A Practical Study Guide

For The

Surgical Technologist Certification Exam
1st Edition

By Joseph J Rios, CST, AS

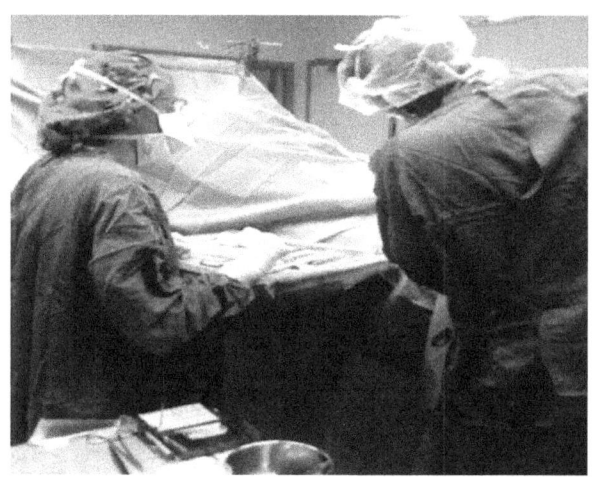

This Study Guide Is Designed For The Preparation Of The Certification

Exam For The Surgical Technologist

This study contains sample questions that have historically been used in prior exams in an effort to familiarize the user in understanding the exam structure.

In addition this study guide contains two (2) 175-question practice exams that will assist the user in understanding the strengths and weaknesses.

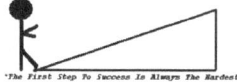

Prepared by Logistical Education Exam Preparation Ltd. (L.E.E.P.Ltd®)
leepltd.com

A Practical Study Guide For The Surgical Technologist Certification Exam

A Practical Study Guide For The Surgical Technologist Certification Exam

© Copyright 2008

ISBN 978-0-615-25074-8

ABOUT THE AUTHOR

Joseph J Rios is a Certified Surgical Technologist with an Associates Degree in Health Science. Joseph was a law enforcement officer with 25 years of experience. He is a certified police instructor and has developed and written a variety of study guides to assist individuals in test preparation techniques. He's followed up these study guides with test preparation seminars. These seminars would vary in length, dependant upon the type of exam the attendees were preparing for. Based on his test preparation techniques his students had a 99% success rate. Statistically students who have followed his "A Practical Study Guide For The Surgical Technologist Certification Exam" have had a 80% success rate, coupled with the test preparation seminar have had a 90% success rate. Currently Joseph is the Clinical Coordinator for a CAAHEP approved Surgical Technology program and instructs in the didactic environment.

Introduction

This study guide contains a breakdown of the areas of measurements the certification exam developers require a testing candidate to successfully complete in order to be qualified as a Certified Surgical Technologist. This study contains sample questions that have historically been used in prior exams in an effort to familiarize the user in understanding the exam structure. In addition this study guide contains two (2) 175-question practice exams that will assist the user in understanding their strengths and weaknesses.

The objective of this study guide is to prepare the user in obtaining the best possible score on the Certification Exam for the Surgical Technologist. The breakdowns of the chapters are designed to assist the user in better understanding the topic area the exam developers are measuring. Within the chapters there will be specifically based questions that are designed to simplify the understanding of the topic.

At the end of each chapter there will be a quiz so the user can determine if they need to review this area with their reference material.

At the rear of this study guide the user will find a comprehensive two (2) 175-question simulated certification exams.

This study guide was developed through years of test preparation instruction. Its intended purpose is to be utilized as a guide starting from front to back. The user should refrain from going straight to the simulated certification exam by reading from the front to the back as it was written; the user would have the advantage of finding their weakest areas. This study guide was written as an aid for the reader, not as a replacement of the National Board for Surgical Technologist and Surgical First Assistant's recommended reading material.

A Practical Study Guide For The Surgical Technologist Certification Exam

REFERENCE	AUTHOR
Surgical Technology for the Surgical Technologist 3rd Edition	Paul Price & Kevin Frey
Alexander's Care of the Patient in Surgery	Jane Rothrock
Berry and Kohn's Operating Room Technique	Nancy Marie Phillips
Human Physiology	Rhoades and Pflanzer
Instrumentation for the Operating Room	Shirley M. Tighe
Medical Terminology Systems: A Body Systems Approach	Barbara A. Guylys & Mary Ellen Wedding
Microbiology for the Health Sciences	Gwendolyn R.W. Burton & Paul G. Engelkirk
Principle's of Human Anatomy	Gerard J. Tortora
Surgical Instruments-A Pocket Guide	Maryann Papanier Well & Mary Bradley
Surgical Technology Principles and Practice	Joanne Kotcher Fuller
Taber's Cyclopedic Medical Dictionary	Donald Venes
The Human Body in Health and Disease	Gary A. Thibodeau & Kevin T. Patton
Standards Recommended Practices and Guidelines	AORN
Law & Ethics for Medical Careers	Karen Judson, Carlene Harrison & Sharon Hicks
Pharmacology for the Surgical Technologist	Chris Keegan & Katherine Snyder
Microbiology for the Surgical Technologist	Paul Price & Kevin Frey

A Practical Study Guide For The Surgical Technologist Certification Exam

TABLE OF CONTENTS

About the Author iv

Introduction v

References and Authors vii

Table of Contents viii

Acknowledgement ix

About the Certifying Exam 1

Chapter 1 Peri-Operative Care 4

Chapter 1 Sample Quiz 13

Chapter 1 Sample Quiz Answers and Rational 20

Chapter 2 Additional Duties 24

Chapter 2 Sample Quiz 36

Chapter 2 Sample Quiz Answers and Rational 44

Chapter 3 Basic Science 48

Chapter 3 Sample Quiz 61

Chapter 3 Sample Quiz Answers and Rational 64

Chapter 4 Metric Conversions 67

Chapter 4 Sample Quiz 73

Chapter 4 Sample Quiz Answers and Rational 75

Chapter 5 Exam Preparation Tips 76

Test Taking Strategies 78

Oral Interview 80

Interview Techniques 81

Mock Certification Examination 1 83

Mock Certification Examination Blank Answer Sheet 106

Mock Certification Examination 1 Answers 107

Mock Certification Examination 2 109

Mock Certification Examination Blank Answer Sheet 135

Mock Certification Examination 2 Answers with Reference 136

ACKNOWLEDGMENTS

The author wishes to acknowledge Robert Prince author of <u>Surgical Tech Success Handbook</u>, whose hard work and dedication to the field has given me the desire to make this study guide. I would also like to acknowledge my wife Eunice, sons Joseph and Michael, daughters Mayah, and Emily for their support, and patience.

ABOUT THE CERTIFYING EXAM

This study guide is designed to assist the reader in identifying their weak areas in a simulated format.

The National Certifying Examination for Surgical Technologists is constructed based on the content outline, using questions from the surgical technologist item bank, and job analysis.

The percentage assigned to each area of the content outline determines how many questions from that area appear on the exam. No two examinations are the exactly the same. Each exam is weighted through percentages, which means that if a certain area of content must contain 60% i.e. Peri-Operative Patient Care and this is percentage is further broken down i.e. 17% Pre-Operative Preparation that this means that the amount of questions within the 60% Peri-Operative Patient Care will contain 17% Pre-Operative Preparation questions.

The content of the exam is based on tasks performed by the Certified Surgical Technologist nationwide. A "job analysis" survey of surgical technologists was conducted to identify the specific tasks to the work of surgical technologists nationwide. A job analysis is used to develop the exam.

A Practical Study Guide For The Surgical Technologist Certification Exam

Although the distribution of items in each content area is similar to the certification exam some questions may be very general and could apply to any type of surgery. Questions apply to the basic fundamental knowledge area. A better break down of the exam is as follows:

(The following is an estimate on the break down of the certification examination based on 175-question exam.)

Perioperative Patient Care 60%

    17% Pre-operative Preparations = approximately 30 questions

    37% Intra-operative Procedures = approximately 65 questions

    6% Post-operative Patient Care = approximately 10 questions

Additional Duties 11%

    3% Administration and Personnel = approximately 5 questions

    8% Sterilization and Maintenance = approximately 14 questions

Basic Science 29%

    17% Anatomy and Physiology   = approximately 30 questions

    6% Microbiology   = approximately 10 questions

    6 % Pharmacology   =approximately 11 questions

A Practical Study Guide For The Surgical Technologist Certification Exam

Chapter 1

I. Peri-Operative Care (60%)

A. Pre-Operative Preparation (17%)

1. Read surgeon's preference card.

2. Verify availability of surgery equipment(e.g., reserve equipment for surgery).

3. Prepare and maintain operating room environment according to surgical procedure (e.g., temperature, lights, suction, and furniture).

4. Review chart (identify and check laboratory results are within normal limits, physician orders, operative consent, allergies, and history and physical).

5. Obtain and apply additional equipment (e.g., pneumatic tourniquet, sequential compression devices, thermoregulatory devices).

6. Don personal protective equipment.

7. Obtain instruments, supplies, and equipment and verify readiness for surgery.

8. Check package integrity of sterile supplies.

9. Open sterile supplies while maintaining aseptic technique.

10. Perform surgical hand scrub, gowning, and gloving.

11. Assemble, inspect, and set up sterile instruments and supplies for surgical procedures.

12. Gown and glove sterile team members.

13. Verify identity of patient and operative site (time out).

14. Drape the patient.

15. Obtain, assemble, and test positioning equipment.

16. Transfer patient to operating room table.

17. Apply patient safety measures
    (e.g., safety strap, elbow protectors, gel pads).

18. Apply patient monitoring devices.

19. Position the patient.

20. Prepare skin for surgery.
    (e.g., hair removal, surgical preparation).

21. Consider the needs of special patient populations
    (e.g., pediatric, geriatric, immune compromised).

The surgical technologist will be measured on their knowledge in areas of surgical attire; gowning; gloving; equipment; supplies; case selection; aseptic technique; surgical counts; and draping. The surgical technologist may be responsible for arranging patient transport, patient positioning; and operating environment. The surgical technologist before donning the sterile gown and gloves must perform a surgical scrub with a chemical antiseptic. Gowns are sterile only in front from chest line to level of sterile field, sleeves from 2" above the elbows to the cuffs. Surgical mask should be changed between every case and handled by the strings only and discarded.

The surgical technologist will be measured on their knowledge of supplies and case selection. The will have to review the function, assembly, use, and care of equipment and surgical supplies. The surgical technologist will need to know the technique that will be used in the surgical procedure in order to gather the instruments; supplies; and equipment needed. The surgical technologist will need to demonstrate the function of accessory surgical equipment, which includes suction systems; lights; ESU (Electro Surgical Unit); Bear Hugger; and tourniquets.

A Practical Study Guide For The Surgical Technologist Certification Exam

Specialty Equipment

1. Lasers

2. Hamonic scalpel

3. Argon-beam coagulator

4. Microscope

5. Video/Monitor/Recorder/Camera

6. Light sources

7. Fiber optic headlight

8. Insufflator

9. Dermatormes

10. Irrigation

11. Cell saver

12. Robotic Arm

Parts of the supplies that the surgical technologist pulls for a case are drapes (knowing what type of procedure each drape is used for); sterile packs; types of sponges; dressing; catheters; tubes and drains. This information can be obtained through the surgeon's preference card or pick sheet.

The surgical technologist has to be familiar with the surgery; the surgeons preference card; and instrumentation.

The surgical technologist is expected to know what supplies are sterile and which are not. The surgical technologist must know each instrument, its classification; it's parts; finishes; care and handling.

The surgical technologist is required to know the principles of asepsis and their application. The surgical technologist will be measured on their knowledge of creating and maintaining a sterile field. The surgical technologist should remember that there is a minimum of three sterile fields to maintain during each surgical procedure.

1. The back table and mayo stand when covered.

2. The surgical field, when the patient is draped.

3. Themselves; the surgeon; and their assistant when gowned and gloved.

The surgical technologist is required to identify contaminants; how they occur; why they occur, and what to do if it does occur.

The surgical technologist will be measured on their knowledge of the surgical scrub. They will need to know what needs to be done prior to the scrub, such as removing all jewelry; wearing PPE (Personal Protection Equipment) and inspecting their skin and nails.

The surgical technologist may be asked about the timed surgical scrub verses the counted brush stroke method of surgical scrub.

The surgical technologist may be asked on the techniques of gowning and gloving oneself and or others; the open gloving technique and the closed glove technique.

B. Intra-Operative Procedures (37%)

1. Provide intra-operative assistance under the direction of the surgeon.

2. Count instrument pre- and intra-operatively with circulator.

3. Identify instruments by:

a) function

b) application

c) classification

4. Count sponges and sharps pre- and intra-operatively with circulator.

5. Anticipate the steps of surgical procedures.

6. Differentiate among the various methods and applications of hemostasis (e.g., mechanical, thermal, chemical).

7. Specify methods of operative exposure.

8. Place and secure retractors.

9. Verify with surgeon the correct type and/or size of implantable devices.

10. Pass instruments and supplies during surgery.

11. Irrigate, suction, and sponge operative site.

12. Monitor and maintain aseptic technique throughout the procedure.

13. Assemble, test and operate specialty equipment during surgery.

14. Utilize the following specialty equipment:

a) argon beam coagulators

b) computer navigation systems

c) thermal ablation

d) robotic technology

e) laser technology

f) ultrasound technology (e.g., harmonic scalpel, phacoemulsification)

g) endoscopic technology

15. Verify and label medications and solutions at the sterile field.

16. Mix medications and solutions at the sterile field.

17. Calculate and report the amount of medications and solutions used.

18. Monitor and maintain adequate supplies and solutions.

19. Prepare drains, catheters, and tubing for insertion.

20. Verify, prepare, and label specimen(s).

21. Observe patient's intra-operative status (e.g., monitor color of blood, onset of blood loss, monitor position of patient during procedure).

22. Apply thermal surgical techniques and safety precautions as directed by the surgeon (e.g., cryo-surgery, laser surgery, ESU).

23. Prepare suture materials.

24. Cut suture material as directed.

25. Identify appropriate usage of sutures/needles and stapling devices.

26. Provide assistance with internal stapling devices.

27. Provide assistance with stapling skin tissue.

28. Perform appropriate actions during an emergency.

29. Initiate preventative and/or corrective actions in potentially hazardous situations.

30. Perform video recording and/or still photography or procedures (e.g., endoscopic).

31. Connect and activate drains to suction apparatus.

32. Prepare and apply sterile dressing.

33. Assist in the placement of wound drainage systems.

34. Apply casts, splints, braces, and similar devices.

C. Post-Operative Procedures (6%)

1. Evaluate patient immediately post-operative and report findings (e.g., bleeding at surgical site, hematoma).

2. Transfer patient from operating table to stretcher.

3. Remove drapes from patient.

4. Perform room clean up after surgery.

5. Dispose of contaminated waste and drapes after surgery in compliance with Standard Precautions.

6. Dispose of contaminated sharps after surgery in compliance with Standard Precautions.

7. Return unused supplies and equipment in designated location.

8. Prepare instruments for decontamination and sterilization.

Chapter 1 Sample Quiz

1. The minimum distance a nonsterile person should remain from a sterile field is

    a. 6 inches

    b. 1 foot

    c. 2 feet

    d. 3 feet

2. Each statement regarding OR attire is true except

    a. lab coats worn out of the OR suite should be clean, closed, and knee length

    b. scrub suits are always changed upon re-entry to the OR suite

    c. scrub suits may be worn out of the OR uncovered, if they are changed upon OR re-entry

    d. nonprofessional personnel and visitors must wear approved attire in the OR

3. Crossing the patient's arms across his or her chest may cause

    a. pressure on the ulnar nerve

    b. interference with circulation

    c. postoperative discomfort

    d. interference with respiration

4. Which term indicates low or decreased blood volume

    a. anoxemia

    b. hypovolemia

    c. hypoxia

    d. hypocapnia

5. Which action is the responsibility of the surgical technologist during an intraoperative CPR effort?

    a. remain sterile, and assist as necessary

    b. document all medications given and draw up as necessary

    c. guard sterile field

    d. break scrub and bring defibrillator into the room

6. External cardiac compression

    a. restores and maintains oxygenation

    b. provides pulmonary ventilation

    c. provides oxygen to vital tissues

    d. provides peripheral pulse

7. An acceptable action when drying the hands and arms after the surgical scrub is to

    a. dry from elbow to fingertip

    b. dry thoroughly, cleanest area first

    c. keep the hands and arms close to the body, at waist level

    d. dry one hand and arm thoroughly

8. Which statement regarding the scrub procedure is not true?

    a. reduces the microbial count

    b. leaves an antimircrobial residue

    c. renders the skin aseptic

    d. removes skin oil

9. If used as part of the skin prep, _____ solution should be allowed to dry before electrocautery is used.

    a. Alcohol

    b. Hexachlorophene

    c. Iodophors

    d. Chlorhexidine

10. Surgical mask should be changed:

    a. after each case

    b. every 2 hours

    c. twice a day

    d. after lunch

11. Before donning the sterile gown and gloves, the surgical technologist must:

    a. sterilize the hands and arms

    b. disinfect the hands and arms

    c. perform scrub to surgically clean hands and arms

    d. perform hand wash to surgically clean hands

12. A straight Mayo scissor is classified as a:

    a. Grasping/Holding

    b. Clamping/ occluding

    c. Cutting/dissecting

    d. Retracting/exposing

13. What is the ideal type of instrument finish that should be used during a procedure when laser use is possible?

    a. Stainless steel

    b. Bright

    c. Mirrored

    d. Ebonized

14. Identify the instrument shown below

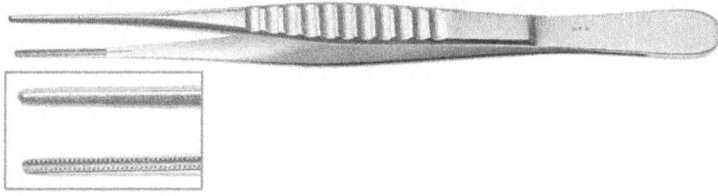

    a. Addson-Brown tissue forceps

    b. Addson-Beckman tissue forceps

    c. Russian tissue forceps

    d. DeBakey tissue forceps

15. Identify the instrument shown below

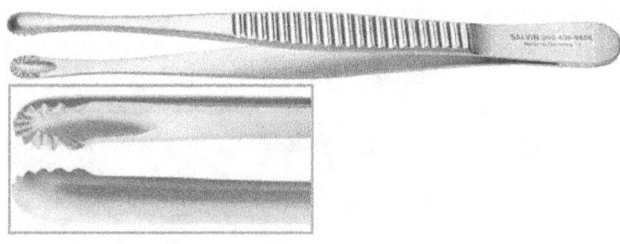

    a. Addson-Brown tissue forceps   c. Russian tissue forceps

    b. Addson-Beckman tissue forceps   d. DeBakey tissue forceps

16. Identify the retractor pictured below

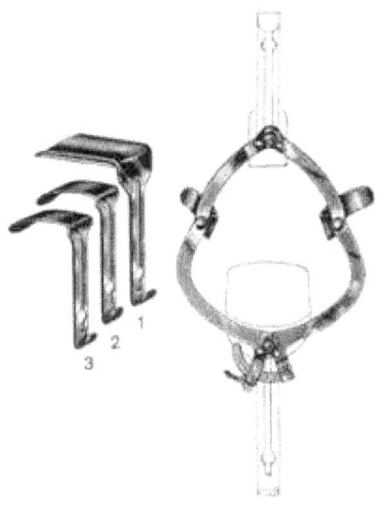

   a. O'Sullivan-O'Connor

   b. Balfour

   c. Gosset

   d. Gellpi

17. What type of instrument is a Lowman?

   a. Orthopedic

   b. Plastic

   c. Cardiovascular

   d. General Surgery

18. Which of the following retractors would not be found in a major orthopedic set?

    a. Bennett

    b. Hohmann

    c. Ragnell

    d. Richardson

19. Exsanguination of a limb before tourniquet inflation is accomplished with wrapping the elevated extremity with

    a. Kling

    b. Esmarch

    c. Stockingette

    d. Webril

20. A regional block that uses the tourniquet is a

    a. Bier block

    b. intrathecal block

    c. peridural block

    d. field block

A Practical Study Guide For The Surgical Technologist Certification Exam

CHAPTER 1 SAMPLE QUIZ
ANSWERS AND RATIONAL

1. **(B)** – All unsterile persons should remain at a minimum of 1 foot from any sterile field. *Surgical Technology for the Surgical Technologist 3rd Edition*

2. **(C)** – All personnel entering the operating room must wear approved, clean attire. Operating room attire is not to be worn, uncovered, out of the operating room. *Surgical Technology for the Surgical Technologist 3rd Edition*

3. **(D)** – Crossing a patient's arms can cause a hindrance of diaphragmatic movement and airway. *Surgical Technology for the Surgical Technologist 3rd Edition*

4. **(B)** – Hypo (low) vol (volume) emia blood. *Medical Terminology Systems: A Body Systems Approach*

5. **(C)** – The surgical technologist remains sterile, guards the sterile field, covers and packs incision, keeps counts, and gives attention to field and surgeon's needs. *Surgical Technology for the Surgical Technologist 3rd Edition*

6. **(C)** – External, cardiac compression maintains circulation, which provides oxygen to the vital body tissues and keeps them viable. *Principle's of Human Anatomy*

7. **(B)** – Dry both hands thoroughly; dry each arm using a rotating motion; do not retrace the area. Bend forward slightly from the waist, and away from the body. The towel should be opened full length. *Surgical Technology for the Surgical Technologist 3rd Edition*

8. **(C)** – The surgical technologist removes skin oil, reduces microbial count, and leaves an antimicrobial residue on the skin. *Surgical Technology for the Surgical Technologist 3rd Edition*

9. **(A)** – Due to the volatile nature of alcohol the skin prep containing alcohol must be allowed to dry prior to the use of the electrocautery; laser or any type of ignition source. *Surgical Technology for the Surgical Technologist 3rd Edition*

10. **(A)** – The surgical mask should be changed after each case. *Surgical Technology for the Surgical Technologist 3rd Edition*

11. **(C)** – Before donning the sterile gown and gloves, the sterile members of the operating room team must perform the surgical scrub with a chemical antiseptic. *Surgical Technology for the Surgical Technologist 3rd Edition*

12. **(C)** – Cutting/dissecting *Surgical Technology for the Surgical Technologist 3rd Edition*

13. **(D)** – When there is a possibility of laser use all instruments should be ebonized or dulled. *Surgical Technology for the Surgical Technologist 3rd Edition*

14. **(D)** – DeBakey tissue forceps a usually for delicate tissues. *Surgical Instruments-A Pocket Guide*

15. **(C)** – Russian tissue forceps take note of the design of the tip. *Surgical Instruments-A Pocket Guide*

16. **(A)** – O'Sullivan- O'Connor *Instrumentation for the Operating Room*

17. **(A)** – A Lowman is a bone holding clamp used primarily for Orthopedic surgery. *Instrumentation for the Operating Room/ Surgical Instruments-A Pocket Guide/ Surgical Technology for the Surgical Technologist 3rd Edition*

18. **(C)** – A Ragnell is a small double ended retractor, primarily utilized in small cases usually to retract skin; delicate vessels; or small tissue. *Berry and Kohn's Operating Room Technique*

19. **(B)** – Exsanguination is the stopping and removal of blood from the extremity's operative site. A Kling and a Webril is a type of dressing; and a Stockingette is impervious covering for the extremity. The Esmarch is a rolled elastic bandage used prior to the tourniquet cuff being inflated. *Surgical Technology for the Surgical Technologist 3rd Edition*

20. **(A)** – A Bier is a regional intravenous injection of a local to an extremity below level of the tourniquet. *Surgical Technology for the Surgical Technologist 3rd Edition*

Chapter 2

II. ADDITIONAL DUTIES (11%)

A. Administrative and Personnel (3%)

1. Revise surgeon's preference card as necessary.

2. Utilize computer technology for:

a) surgeon's preference cards

b) interdepartmental communication

c) continuing education

d) research

3. Follow disaster plan protocol.

4. Recognize safety and environmental hazards (e.g., fire, chemical spill, laser smoke).

5. Follow proper cost containment processes.

6. Apply ethical and legal practices related to surgical patient care.

7. Use interpersonal skills (e.g., listening, diplomacy, responsiveness) and group dynamics.

8. Understand the importance of cultural diversity.

9. Serve as preceptor to perioperative personnel.

B. Equipment Sterilization and Maintenance (8%)

1. Operate sterilizing devices according to manuf. recommendations.

2. Troubleshoot equipment malfunctions.

3. Decontaminate and clean instruments and equipment.

4. Inspect, test, and assemble instruments and equipment.

5. Package and sterilize instruments and equipment.

6. Perform quality assurance functions
(e.g., biological monitoring of sterilization methods).

7. Maintain equipment records and logs
(e.g., Steris, Attest, laser log, steam sterilizers).

The surgical technologist must demonstrate the ability to conduct an inventory of supplies and equipment. A surgical technologist may be called upon to determine what is needed in the operating room environment. They must have a rudimentary knowledge as to what contents are needed in specialty packs; types of suture; tower equipment, and such.

On occasion a surgical technologist may be called upon to manage the materials management department.

The surgical technologist must demonstrate knowledge in the area of sterilization and disinfection. He/she must be able to identify the mechanism utilized in sterilization (e.g. gravity type steam sterilizer; vacuum autoclave; Steris unit). He/She must also demonstrate knowledge in the mechanism used in instrument disinfection; equipment disinfection; the equipment used for disinfection (e.g. ultrasonic washer; Glutaraldehyde; enzymatic cleanser). The surgical technologist will be tested on the methods used for the decontamination of the operating room, and equipment. The surgical technologist must have an understanding of germicidal effects of certain chemicals.

They will also have to demonstrate their knowledge of the environmental factors that influence the growth of microorganism, and what is necessary for infection.

Each surgical technologist will be tested on their knowledge of packaging materials and devices. They will ask the types of folds for certain wrappings, there are several techniques available to wrap an item so it can be presented aseptically. Two of these methods are square fold, also known as the straight method, and the envelope fold, sometimes called the diagonal method. These and other wrapping methods will ensure instruments arrive at their destination in pristine and sterile condition.

Woven textiles

Woven was at one time, the only packaging material available. These are textile (cloth) based and reusable. They can be bleached or unbleached muslin (100%), muslin/polyester blend (50/50), all synthetic blends and the new high density textiles for maximum moisture and bacterial barrier.

Generally, woven textiles (e.g. muslin) are poor moisture and bacterial barriers. Take a cloth wrapper and place water on it to see how quickly the water penetrates. The barrier quality of textiles is usually represented in "thread counts" per square inch. The more threads per square inch, the less space between the fibers, the better the barrier. Therefore, the higher thread count textiles provide better barriers to bacterial. The minimum acceptable thread count for surgical textiles is **140 threads/inch**. To improve the bacterial barrier, two layers of material (ply-wrapper) are sewn together around the edges. The newer textiles have improved moisture and bacterial barriers due to the higher thread counts.

So why use reusable textiles as wrappers and drapes? First, this system is lower in cost, especially if the facility has its own laundry. Since they are reusable, there is no waste generation (it costs money to haul trash away).

The disadvantages include high lint generation; they must be washed, de-linted and inspected before each use. The inspection must be on light table (table with light underneath to see holes/defects).

If defects are identified, they must be patched with heat patch machine placing a patch on both sides of the textile. The defects should not be sewn and no cross-stitching of textiles is permitted because the needle makes additional holes in the wrapper. The overall quality of the wrapper should be assessed each time. Placing multiple heat patches in the same area in not recommended, as steam cannot penetrate through the patches.

The inspection, de-linting, etc. should be performed in a separate room with sufficient air exchanges to keep dust/lint at a minimum and prevent lung illnesses in staff.

Non-woven Materials (man-made)

Non-woven materials (man made) are single use. There are many types including: crepe paper, plastic polymers (e.g. polyolefin), cellulose fibers and washed paper pulp.

The advantages are that they may be cost effective, no laundering is needed and they have small spaces between the fibers (as compared to muslin) so they provide better bacterial/moisture barrier. Many of these products are water repellent (not all).

The disadvantages are that they create waste, can cost more and can tear easily. For quality assurance purposes, a random sampling of wrappers should be inspected when a new box is opened. The products are available in single ply or double ply.

Wrapping Techniques

There are two basic techniques; the square fold and the envelope fold. Usually, the square fold is used for large sets while the envelope fold is used for most other items.

The single ply material and reusable textiles requires two separate wrappers be applied sequentially (one wrapper applied at a time). This is called "sequential wrapping". The double ply material only requires one piece of packaging material because it has two wrappers bonded at least one end. This is called "simultaneous wrapping".

Packaging Principles

You need to select the correct size wrapper- not too big or too small. When wrapping the first fold should completely cover the item inside the pack. Apply the wrapper secure enough to keep contents secure but loose enough to allow air removal and sterilant penetration. A wrapper that is too loose can cause microorganisms and dust to enter the pack. When a package is wrapped, it is important to understand how the end user will open the package; the opening should be on the top; not the bottom.

Item's, which cannot be used to secure packs, includes staples, pins, rubber bands, paper clips or anything sharp that can damage the packaging material. Always use sterilization tape specific to the sterilization process being used.

Pouches

Pouches (also peel pouch, visi peel) have a material composition of paper and mylar (clear side) or all plastic (Tyvek - polyethylene). Tyvek pouches are all plastic and therefore cannot be used in steam or they melt. They are only intended for low temperature sterilization processes.

The placement of items inside pouch is critical. It is recommended to leave at least a one-inch space around the device. The end of device (finger rings) should be facing the end where the pouch will be opened.

It is important to select the correct size pouch; if the pouch is too large, the item can get damaged from moving around; if the pouch is too small, the seals on the pouch can rupture during sterilization.

NOTE; pouches are intended for single, light weight items!

Pouches can be closed by heat sealing - (use the heat sealer (temperature and pressure) according to the sealer manufacturer) or self-sealing (make sure there are no creases, crevices in folds). All air should be expelled from the pouch before sealing to prevent pressure on the seals during and after sterilization.

Double pouching is not required. If it is necessary to contain small items, the inside pouch must lay flat inside outer pouch with

NO FOLDING OVER THE ENDS!

Plastic Films (Dust or Sterility Maintenance Covers)

Plastic films (sterility maintenance covers) are effective to keep out moisture and contaminates from sterile packages. They are applied to traditional packaging (textiles of non-wovens) after sterilization. They must be applied correctly and selection of the correct size bag is important. Before applying, the item must be completely cool (about 1 hour after sterilization). Never apply a dust cover to a warm/hot tray because condensate can form inside.) When applying the dust cover, expel all the air from the bag before sealing.

Make sure your hands have been washed before starting the sealing process or wear gloves to prevent adding more microbes inside the bag.

Dust covers must be a specific thickness (2-3 millimeters). Thickness' of less than 2 mils can have defects which can cause contamination. Only products labeled, as dust covers should be used for this purpose.) Dust covers can be closed by heat sealing - (use the heat sealer (temperature and pressure) according to the sealer manufacturer's instructions for heat sealing plastic bags) or self-sealing (make sure there are no creases, crevices in folds). Verify the seal has no defects.

__Rigid Containers__

Rigid containers are commonly used today to protect instruments in transport/storage. The components of the system include a top, base, inner basket, filter retention rings/plates, etc. Containers must be cleaned, inspected and sterilized according to the manufacturer's instructions. Containers can have single use filters or a valve system. Some offer a location for a load card to place the lot control number sticker. Always use the filters recommended by the container manufacturer. Generally, remove/discard the filters after each use and remove the load card. Containers must be disassembled and washed (not wiped) after each use.

For quality control, rigid containers should be inspected each time they are used. Check that the gasket is free of defects; that there are no dents in the container; that the lid fits correctly and the filter retention plate fits snugly (filter cannot remove around). Some containers have valves (no filters); you need information on the frequency of valve replacement.

To keep the container closed and to assure no open opened the container after sterilization; containers require a locking mechanism at each end. It is important to make sure the locks are present. Some locks have a chemical indicator printed on them.

Chemical Indicators

All items being sterilized must have an internal and external chemical indicator. The external chemical indicator (CI) simply identifies an item that has been through a process from one that has not. Internal chemical indicators play an important role in sterility assurance. In order for the CI to turn color, the sterilant must make contact with the CI. If air is present or if there is insufficient sterilant, the color change will be incomplete or not take place at all. It is important to know and understand the correct color change for the CI being used and to always verify that the correct color change took place.

The CI should always be placed in the geometric center of the pack or tray since this is the most difficult location for the sterilant to reach.

The only exception is with rigid containers where the CI should be placed in two opposite corners since corners are usually where air gets trapped in containers. Multi-level trays should have a CI placed on each level.

Packaging uses

The recommended sterilization processes for the various types of packaging materials are:

Muslin/textiles - steam, ETO, dry heat (if not in excess of 425F)

1. Peel packs - steam, ETO

2. Paper wrap (crepe paper) - steam, ETO

3. Tyvek - ETO, low temperature gas plasma, NO STEAM

4. Polyolefin (plastic) wrap (e.g. Kimguard) - steam, ETO, LTGP

Package Labels:

Whenever an item is packaged, it should be identified with the department, name of the device and the initials of the preparer. This helps to track quality issues. Writing should always be done on autoclave tape, not on the packaging material. It is recommended that non-toxic markers that will not bleed or smear be used. Use of lead pencils or ball-point pens is not recommended as they may contain toxins which can be distributed in the sterilizer. It is not recommended to write on the packaging material because the pen can possibly damage the fibers of the packaging. On peel pouch material, writing can be made on the clear side, not the plastic side.

Packaging Closures:

Autoclave tape is the recommended closure for wrapped sets. Masking tape should never be used because it was not intended to be sterilize and will not differentiate a set that has been in a sterilizer from one that has not. Use as little tape as possible so the end user can easily get into the package; excessive tape can hamper correct opening of the tray.

Chapter 2 Sample Quiz

1. A wet-vacuum detergent with a disinfection solution is used

    a. to sterilize operating room floors

    b. only when patient has aids

    c. at the end of each procedure

    d. never used in the operating room

2. Safe temperature for the operating is?

    a. 49° to 56° F

    b. 56° to 67° F

    c. 60° to 75° F

    d. 80° to 85° F

3. Operating rooms have air pressure _____ corridor air.

   a. that constantly adjusts to

   b. greater than

   c. less than

   d. equal to

4. The required number of air exchanges per hour in an operating room is?

   a. 5 – 10

   b. 10 – 15

   c. 15 - 20

   d. 20 –25

5. If an adult patient refuses a blood transfusion, the hospital should

   a. give blood on in an emergency

   b. perform no operation that requires a transfusion

   c. ask next of kin

   d. give no blood

6. Lead is the best shield against

   a. Gamma rays

   b. barium

   c. co2 laser

   d. barium

   e. elecrocautery

7. Nonexplosive proof of electrical plugs should placed

   a. above baseboards

   b. a minimum height of 5 feet

   c. near anesthesia cart

   d. a minimum higher of 4 feet

8. Between operations, decontaminatin of wall involves washing

    a. only from the floor up 3ft level with

    b. all walls from the floor up to a 4th level with solution

    c. all walls with disinfectant solution

    d. only areas that have been splashed with blood or organic debris

9. The surgeon returns a broken needle; the surgical technologist should immediately:

    a. inform consent

    b. ask for an ex-ray

    c. change to new needle and say

    d. tell the circulator

10. A dimly light and quiet room is

    a. Not recommended as pre-op area

    b. The surgeon's preference

    c. Recommended as a pre-op environment

    d. D. not necessary for surgery

11. If hemostat is left in a patient who received an appendectomy, what would the legal charge be?

    a. Res ipsa loguitor

    b. Misdemeanor

    c. Intentional tort

    d. Extension doctrine

12. If a countable item is lost, what is done first?

    a. Inform the surgeon

    b. A count is repeated immediately

    c. Order x-ray of the operative site

    d. In form the circulator

13. In a true surgical emergency, which counting procedure is followed?

    a. do all required counts

    b. only initial count is required

    c. only final count is required

    d. omit count, indicate on the operative record

14. Of the following information, what is not necessary to be in patient's chart?

    a. patient's MR number

    b. chest film

    c. signed informed consent

    d. patient's date of birth

15. Furniture and equipment should be damp-dusted.

    a. only after last case of the day

    b. only if contaminated with blood

    c. after every case with a disinfectant

    d. after every case with an antiseptic

16. The parents of a minor requires emergency surgery and they can not be found, the consent form

    a. may be waived

    b. can be signed by the surgeon

    c. can be signed by Operating Room Director and Surgeon

    d. can be discussed with anesthesiologist

17. Traffic in the Operating Room should be

    a. no different than any other area of the hospital

    b. reduced to prevent contamination of sterile field

    c. reduced to avoid making the patient nervous

    d. increased to prevent delay of procedure

18. The operative record must include all of the following except

    a. plan for therapeutic and follow-up care

    b. preoperative skin prep method

    c. position and position aids used

    d. location of the grounding pad

19. Performing surgery on a patient without a signed consent is

    a. slander

    b. assault

    c. defamation

    d. battery

20. A patient is burned from improper placement of the electrosurgical ground pad whose primary legal responsibility is it?

    a. anesthesiologist

    b. Operating Room Supervisor

    c. Circulator

    d. Surgeon

A Practical Study Guide For The Surgical Technologist Certification Exam

CHAPTER 2 SAMPLE QUIZ
ANSWERS AND RATIONAL

1. **(c)** Ideally the operating room floor should always be disinfected using a wet-vacuum detergent with a disinfection solution. The operating room floor will always be cleaned with a disinfection solution when a wet-vacuum is not available. *Surgical Technology for the Surgical Technologist 3rd Edition*

2. **(c)** The safe temperature for the operating room to aid in the prevention of microbial growth is 60° F – 75° F (15° C - 23° C) *Surgical Technology for the Surgical Technologist 3rd Edition*

3. **(b)** The air pressure in an operating room is greater than the exterior corridors, this is to prevent airborne contaminates from enter the operating room. *Surgical Technology for the Surgical Technologist 3rd Edition*

4. **(d)** A patient has the legal authority to refuse a blood transfusion and the hospital is required to abide by their decision. *Surgical Technology Principles and Practice/ Surgical Technology for the Surgical Technologist 3rd Edition*

5. **(c)** The air in the operating room setting is required to exchange 15 – 20 times per hour to remove airborne particles from the environment. *Surgical Technology for the Surgical Technologist 3rd Edition*

6. **(a)** For gamma rays and x rays, lead is a particularly effective shield. *Standards Recommended Practices and Guidelines/ Surgical Technology for the Surgical Technologist 3rd Edition*

7. **(b)** A required standard in the operating room setting is that all nonexplosive proof electrical plugs should be a minimum of 5 feet from the floor. *Surgical Technology for the Surgical Technologist 3rd Edition/Standards Recommended Practices and Guidelines*

8. **(d)** Decontamination of the operating room after each case is essential and that all walls that have or may have been exposed to bodily fluids be washed and disinfected. *Microbiology for the Surgical Technologist/ Surgical Technology Principles and Practice*

9. **(a)** Inform the surgeon, the surgeon may know where to find it and it also prevents the surgeon from sharps injury. If the needle is not located an x-ray will be called in an effort to locate the broken piece of needle. *Surgical Technology Principles and Practice/ Standards Recommended Practices and Guidelines*

10. **(c)** The environment setting for pre-op is dimly lighted and quiet room so the level of anxiety can be lowed with the assistance of a sedative. *Berry and Kohn's Operating Room Technique*

11. **(a)** Res ipsa loquitor translates to "the thing speaks for itself". *Surgical Technology for the Surgical Technologist 3rd Edition*

12. **(b)** As stated a counted is repeated immediately, to ensure there was a miscount. *Surgical Technology for the Surgical Technologist 3rd Edition/ Berry and Kohn's Operating Room Technique*

13. **(d)** In a true emergency a count is secondary to immediate surgical intervention. It must be noted on the operative record. *Surgical Technology for the Surgical Technologist 3rd Edition/ Berry and Kohn's Operating Room Technique*

14. **(b)** A patient's MR (Medical Record) number is required in the chart, along with the patients name; date of birth and signed consent form. *Law & Ethics for Medical Careers*

15. **(c)** An operating room damp dusted with disinfecting solution first thing in the morning, and after each case thereafter. *Surgical Technology for the Surgical Technologist 3rd Edition*

16. **(a)** As in this answer you are looking for the most correct answer, which is "the consent form may be waived." *Law & Ethics for Medical Careers/ Surgical Technology for the Surgical Technologist 3rd Edition*

17. **(b)** Traffic movement in the operating room increases the risk of contamination of sterile field. It is for this reason all traffic is kept to a minimum. *Surgical Technology for the Surgical Technologist 3rd Edition*

18. **(a)** The patient's operative chart must contain the preoperative skin prep; position of positioning aids used and the location of

the grounding pad. Post Anesthesia Care Unit personnel perform documenting of the plan for therapeutic and follow-up care. *Standards Recommended Practices and Guidelines/ Law & Ethics for Medical Careers*

19. **(d)** Any action taken on a patient without their signed written consent is considered battery under the law. *Law & Ethics for Medical Careers/ Surgical Technology for the Surgical Technologist 3rd Edition*

20. **(c)** The circulator is responsible for the placement of the grounding pad. *Surgical Technology for the Surgical Technologist 3rd Edition/ Standards Recommended Practices and Guidelines*

Chapter 3

III. BASIC SCIENCE (29%)

A. Anatomy and Physiology (17%)

1. Use appropriate medical terminology and abbreviations.

2. Demonstrate knowledge of the following anatomical systems as they relate to the surgical procedure:

a) cardiovascular

b) digestive

c) endocrine

d) integumentary

e) lymphatic

f) muscular

g) nervous

h) peripheral vascular

i) reproductive

j) respiratory

k) sensory

l) skeletal

m) urinary

3. Demonstrate knowledge of human physiology as it relates to the surgical procedure for the following systems:

a) cardiovascular

b) digestive

c) endocrine

d) integumentary

e) lymphatic

f) muscular

g) nervous

h) peripheral vascular

i) reproductive

j) respiratory

k) sensory

l) skeletal

m) urinary

4. Identify the following surgical pathologies:

a) abnormal anatomy

b) disease processes

c) fractures

d) malignancies

B. Microbiology (6%)

1. Apply the following principles of surgical microbiology to operative practice:

a) classification and pathogenesis of microorganisms

b) factors influencing wound healing (e.g., condition of patient, wound type)

c) infection control procedures (e.g., aseptic technique)

d) principles of tissue handling (e.g., Halsted principles, tissue manipulation methods, traction/counter traction)

e) stages of, and factors influencing wound healing

f) surgical wound classification.

2. Identify and address factors that can influence an infectious process.

C. Surgical Pharmacology (6%)

1. Apply the following principles of surgical pharmacology to operative practice:

a) anesthesia related agents and medications

b) blood and fluid replacement

c) complications from drug interactions (e.g., malignant hyperthermia)

d) methods of anesthesia administration (e.g., general, local, block)

e) types, uses, action, and interactions of drugs and solution (e.g., hemostatic agents, antibiotics, IV)

Anatomy and Physiology

I. Integumentary System:

A. The surgical technologist must identify the three major regions of skin

    1. epidermis (outer epithelial layers)

    2. dermis (middle connective tissue region)

    3. subcutaneous (hypodermis) (deeper adipose region)

B. The surgical technologist must be able to identify the epidermal strata in skin

    1. stratum corneum (outermost portion - keratinized)

    2. stratum spinosum

    3. stratum lucidum (only on palms & soles)

    4. stratum granulosum

    5. stratum basale (also called germinativum - highest mitotic activity)

C. The surgical technologist must be able to identify these integumentary cells and structures (know the **functions of each**)

    1. keratinocytes,

    2. melanocytes,

    3. adipocytes,

    4. fibroblasts,

    5. merkle cells,

    6. pacinian corpuscles,

    7. arrector pili,

    8. sebaceous glands,

        a. differentiate "eccrine" from "apocrine" sweat glands.

    9. sudoriferous glands,

    10. papillary region,

    11. reticular region,

D. The surgical technologist must identify the following forms of skin cancer

    1. basal cell carcinoma (BCC)

    2. squamous cell carcinoma (SCC)

    3. malignant melanoma

4. identify the ABCDs of examining skin cancer lesions

    a. A- assymeteric shape

    b. B- border that is irregular or diffuse

    c. C- color that is pearly or multicolored

    d. D- diameter larger than 5mm

E. The surgical technologist must demonstrate knowledge of the characteristics of 1st, 2nd, and 3rd degree burns

    1. be able to use the "Rule of Nines" to estimate body surface area involved in burns

II. Anatomical directions and orientation:

A. The surgical technologist must be able to identify major body structures with proper directional terminology

    1. superior(cephalic or cranial)/inferior(caudal)

    2. anterior(ventral)/posterior(dorsal)

    3. lateral/medial(mesial)

    4. contralateral/ipsilateral

    5. proximal/distal

    6. superficial/deep

B. The surgical technologist must be able to identify the major body cavities & structures

    1. cranial cavity

    2. vertebral cavity

    3. thoracic cavity

        a. diaphragm

        b. pleural cavity

        c. pericardial cavity

        d. mediastinum

    4. abdominal cavity

    5. serous membranes

C. Be able to locate and identify the major abdominopelvic regions

    1. R/L hypochondriac regions

    2. epigastric/hypogastric regions

    3. R/L lumbar regions

    4. R/L iliac(inguinal) regions

    5. umbilical region

D. Define: radiography, CT, PET, MRI and ultrasound

III. Osteology (bone histology)

A. Identify the major functions of the skeletal system:

B. Be able to use proper anatomical terms describing bones:

    1. diaphysis

    2. epiphysis

    3. metaphysis

    4. epiphyseal plate

    5. articular cartilage

    6. periosteum & endosteum

    7. compact & spongy bone

C. Identify the function of bone cells:

    1. osteoprogenitor

    2. osteoblast

    3. osteocyte

    4. osteoclast

D. Describe the two major processes of bone formation:

    1. endochondral (long bone formation)

    2. intramembraneous (flat bone formation)

E. Describe the process of bone remodeling & repair:

  1. cells involved

  2. factors affecting bone remodeling

F. Describe the role of bone tissue and cells in calcium homeostasis:

  1. Describe the effects of these hormones on bone tissue

    a. parathyroid hormone

    b. calcitonin

    c. calcitriol (vitamin D)

    d. estrogen

    e. growth hormone

    f. insulin

IV. Skeleton (know all axial vs. appendicular bones):

  A. The surgical technologist must have the knowledge to demonstrate the location and be able to identify the bones of the skull (cranial & facial bones)

B. Locate and identify the four major sutures of the skull

    1. coronal

    2. sagittal

    3. squamosal

    4. lambdoidal

C. Identify the following and state their significance...

    1. fontanelles

    2. microcephaly

    3. paranasal and mastoid sinuses

    4. deviated nasal septum

    5. damaged cribrifrom plate

    6. cleft palate

D. Locate and identify the bones of the spinal column

    1. cervical vertebrae (7)

        a. what are "spinal nerves"?

    2. thoracic vertebrae (12)

    3. lumbar vertebrae (5)

    4. sacrum (1)

    5. coccyx (1)

E. Identify the following and state their significance...

    1. normal spinal curvatures

    2. scoliosis

    3. kyphosis

    4. lordosis

    5. spina bifida

F. Identify the bones of the pelvic girdle

    1. distinguish between male and female pelvic bones

V. Articulations:

A. The surgical technologist must have the knowledge basis for structural & functional classifications of joints:

    1. structural classes

      a. fibrous

      b. cartilaginous

      c. synovial

    2. functional classes

      a. synarthrosis

      b. amphiarthrosis

      c. diarthrosis

B. Describe the synovial capsule structure including:

    1. inner and outer membranes

    2. state the source, composition and functions of synovial fluid

    3. what function do synovial phagocytes serve?

    4. articular cartilage surfaces

    5. accessory ligaments

    6. menisci

    7. bursae

a. how are bursae similar to synovial cavities?

b. where does the fluid in the bursae come from?

C. Shoulder (glenohumeral) joint:

    1. locate and identify the rotator cuff muscles

      a. supraspinatus

      b. infraspinatus

      c. suscapular

      d. teres minor

D. Knee (tibiofemoral) joint:

    1. locate and identify the bones and major ligaments of the knee

      a. patellar & quadriceps femoris

      b. lateral & medial collaterals

      c. anterior & posterior cruciates

    2. locate and identify the medial (C) and lateral (O) menisci

E. Arthritic Disorders:

    1. The surgical technologist must have the knowledge of the causes, typical manifestations, and treatments of the following...

      a. rheumatoid arthritis

b. osteoarthritis

c. gouty arthritis

2. describe "arthroscopy" and "arthroplasty"

A Practical Study Guide For The Surgical Technologist Certification Exam

Chapter 3 Sample Quiz

1. ____ is the multiplication of organisms in tissue.
   a. Nosocomial
   b. Infection
   c. cross contamination
   d. Culture

2. *Escherichia coli* normally resides in the lumen of the ____.
   a. Esophagus
   b. Trachea
   c. intestine
   d. urethra

3. Bacilli are typically found to be in the shape of a ____.
   a. Spiral
   b. Round
   c. L form
   d. Rod

4. In which phase of healing does a wound undergo a slow, sustained increase in tissue tensile strength?
   a. Lag
   b. Proliferation
   c. maturation
   d. inflammatory response

5. In the proliferation phase, which of the following forms into fiber that give the wound approximately 25% to 30% of its original tensile strength?
   a. Leukocytes
   b. Collagen
   c. basal cells
   d. fibroblasts

6. Which of the following does NOT belong to the category of malignant neoplasm?
   a. Glioblastoma
   b. colon cancer
   c. breast cancer
   d. endometriosis

7. Which is a common physiological factor in the elderly?
   a. increased cardiac output
   b. increased heart rate
   c. decreased coronary artery blood flow
   d. increased coronary artery blood flow

8. Anesthesia affects the normal ____ and physiological process of insulin.
   a. metabolic
   b. caloric intake
   c. glucose
   d. Serum

9. Immediate operative intervention is performed on the pregnant patient for the following emergency procedures EXCEPT:
   a. appendicitis
   b. competent cervical os
   c. traumatic injury
   d. ectopic pregnancy

10. During abdominal procedures on obese patients, what procedure might additionally be performed due to newly identified pathology?
    a. pancreatectomy
    b. Whipple
    c. cholecystectomy
    d. splenectomy

11. During birth, the most common bone fracture is of the ____.
    a. radius
    b. fibula
    c. clavicle
    d. skull

12. Drugs with a high potential to cause psychological and/or physical dependence and abuse are called ____.
    a. over the counter
    b. Chemical
    c. prescription
    d. controlled substances

13. Demerol, Sublimaze, Sufenta, and Alfenta are examples of ____.
    a. Opioids
    b. dissociative agents
    c. narcotic antagonists
    d. hypnotic agents

14. Antiemetic agents are used to prevent ____.
    a. Bleeding
    b. Nausea
    c. clotting
    d. hypotension

15. Which agents selectively interrupt the associative pathways of the brain?
    a. opioids
    b. dissociative
    c. induction
    d. tranquilizers

16. Patient position, and agent baricity can influence the effect of ____.
    a. nerve plexus
    b. local anesthetic
    c. spinal anesthetic
    d. caudal block

17. Nerve plexus block, Bier block, spinal block, and epidural block are common types of ____.
    a. local infiltration
    b. monitored anesthesia
    c. cryoanesthesia
    d. regional blockade

18. Calcium chloride is an example of an electrolyte replacement drug used to ____.
    a. fight against malignant hyperthermia
    b. fight against malignant hypothermia
    c. stimulate the myocardium
    d. relax the myocardium

19. Which class of surgical wounds has the highest rate of infection?
    a. I
    b. II
    c. III
    d. IV

20. The final wound classification is assigned when ____.
    a. an incision is made
    b. a wound is drained
    c. inflammation is present
    d. the procedure is finished

A Practical Study Guide For The Surgical Technologist Certification Exam
CHAPTER 3 SAMPLE QUIZ
ANSWERS AND RATIONAL

1. **(B)** –Infectious organisms multiply throughout the tissue. *Surgical Technology for the Surgical Technologist 3rd Edition*

2. **(C)** – *Escherichia coli* normally resides in the lumen of the intestine *Microbiology for the Health Sciences*

3. **(D)** – The common shape of the bacilli is rod shaped. *Microbiology for the Health Sciences*

4. **(C)** – During the Maturation phase a wound undergoes a slow, sustained increase in tissue tensile strength. *Human Physiology*

5. **(B)** – In the proliferation phase, collagen forms into fibers that give the wound approximately 25% to 30% of its original tensile strength. *Human Physiology*

6. **(D)** – Endometriosis is a common medical condition characterized by growth beyond or outside the uterus of tissue resembling endometrium, the tissue that normally lines the uterus. *The Human Body in Health and Disease*

7. **(C)** – Elderly patients with acute coronary syndromes suffer higher mortality and more morbidity than their younger counterparts because they have higher prevalence of cardiac risk factors. *Human Physiology*

8. **(A)**–Anesthesia affects the normal metabolic and physiological process of insulin. *Surgical Technology for the Surgical Technologist 3rd Edition*

9. **(B)** – Competent cervical os *Principle's of Human Anatomy*

10. **(C)** – Obesity constitutes a clear risk factor for cholelithiasis, especially if it is associated abdominal surgery. Prophylactic cholecystectomy is indicated in biliopancreatic diversions due to the high incidence of postoperative cholelithiasis. *The Human Body in Health and Disease*

11. **(C)** – The most common bone injury sustained in birth is fracture of the clavicle, which is always a risk when a large baby is delivered. *Surgical Technology for the Surgical Technologist 3rd Edition*

12. **(D)** – Drugs with a high potential to cause psychological and/or physical dependence and abuse are called controlled substances *Pharmacology for the Surgical Technologist*

13. **(A)** – An opioid is a chemical substance that has a morphine-like action in the body. The main use is for pain relief. *Pharmacology for the Surgical Technologist*

14. **(B)** – Antiemetic agents are used to prevent nausea. *Pharmacology for the Surgical Technologist*

15. **(B)** – Dissociative Agents-selectively interrupt the associative pathways of the brain. Appear awake but unaware of surroundings. *Pharmacology for the Surgical Technologist*

16. **(C)** – Patient position and agent baricity can influence the effect of spinal anesthetic *Surgical Technology for the Surgical Technologist 3rd Edition*

17. **(D)** – Nerve plexus block, Bier block, spinal block, and epidural block are common types of regional blockade. *Surgical Technology for the Surgical Technologist 3rd Edition*

18. **(C)** – Calcium chloride can be used as aid in management of the acute symptoms in lead colic; in cardiac resuscitation, particularly after open heart surgery. Parenteral calcium can be used when epinephrine has failed to improve weak or ineffective myocardial contractions. *Surgical Technology for the Surgical Technologist 3rd Edition*

19. **(D)** – Class IV/Dirty or Infected Wounds--old traumatic wounds with retained or devitalized tissue and those that involve existing clinical infection or perforated viscera. This definition suggests that the organisms causing postoperative infection were present in the wound before the surgical procedure
Standards Recommended Practices and Guidelines

20. **(A)** – The final wound classification is assigned when the procedure is finished.
Surgical Technology for the Surgical Technologist 3rd Edition

METRIC CONVERSIONS

The surgical technologist must be able to demonstrate their knowledge of metric conversions. All measurements within the operating room environment are either conducted under the metric system or French measurement system.

Metric Conversion Chart

Abbreviation	Definition
ML, ml	Milliliter
cc	Cubic centimeter
g	Gram
mg	Milligram
gr	Grain
mcg	Microgram
mm	Millimeter
cm	Centimeter
In.	Inch
ft.	Foot
lbs.	Pounds
kg	Kilograms
Tsp	Teaspoon
Tbsp	Tablespoon

GRAM	G	WEIGHT
METER	M	LENGTH
LITER	L	VOLUME

Conversion Factors

UNITS OF VOLUME (LITER)		UNITS OF SOLIDS	
* 1 cc	1 ml	* 1 g	1000 mg
* 1 liter	1000ml	* 1 mg	1000 mcg
1 L	100 centiliters	1 g	100 centigrams
1 L	10 deciliters	1 g	10 decigrams
1 dekaliter	10 L	1 dekagram	10 g
1 hectoliter	100 L	1 hectogram	100 g
1 kiloliter	1000 L	1 kilogram	1000 g
LIQUID MEASUREMENT		WEIGHT	
METRIC	APOTHECARY	METRIC	APOTHECARY
* 1000ml	1 quart	30 g	1 oz
* 500 ml	1 pint	15 g	4 drams
* 30 ml	1 fluid oz	1 g	15 grains
1 ml	15 OR 16 minims	0.5g	7 ½ gr.
0.06 ml	1 minim	* 60 mg	1 gr.
		30 mg	½ gr.
		1 mg	1/60 gr.
OTHER			
METRIC	MISC.	METRIC/misc	MISC.
* 5 cc	1 TSP	2.5 cm	1 in.
* 15 cc's	1 TBSP	12 in.	1 ft
240 cc's	1 CUP	10 mm	1 cm
* 1 kg	2.2 lbs		

* Memorize

Metric Conversion Chart-Directions

Practice problem:

What is the conversion factor for grams to milligrams?

Rule: When referring to the "conversion factor," look at the chart provided and find the units mentioned. There should be two numbers listed. The conversion factor is the number other than 1.

Example: What is the conversion factor for grams to milligrams?

1 g = 1000 mg (from table)

So the conversion factor is **1000**

To convert *from* a smaller unit *to* a larger unit, **Divide** by the conversion factor

To convert *from* a larger unit *to* a smaller unit, **Multiply** by the conversion factor

Practice problem:

The physician has ordered Tylenol 1g by mouth now.

Our on hand supply is Tylenol 500 mg tablets.

Rule: If the unit of the physicians order and the unit of your supply are different you must convert the physicians order so that both are the same unit (either grams, milligrams, etc.). See box above for directions.

Example: The physician has ordered Tylenol 1g by mouth to be given now.

Our on hand supply is Tylenol 500 mg tablets.

1. Change the 1gram to __?__ milligrams

2. Find the conversion factor from the table (1000)

3. We are converting from a larger unit to a smaller unit so we must multiply by the conversion factor. Formula & example follow:

A Practical Study Guide For The Surgical Technologist Certification Exam
MD order x Conversion factor = "new" MD order with new unit title

1 g x 1000 = 1000 mg

How do I know what is the larger unit? See the boxes below.

Example in $	$1000	$100	$10	$1	.10¢	.01¢	.001¢	.000001¢
Placement	THOUSANDS	HUNDREDS	TENS	ONES	TENTHS	HUNDREDTHS	THOUSANDTHS	MILLIONTHS
Metric Term	KILO	HECTO	DEKA	SINGLE UNIT	DECI	CENTI	MILLI	MICRO
Abbreviation	k	h	dk	g, L, or m	d	c	m	mc

Add g, L, or m after the abbreviation to indicate weight, liquid, or length.
Example: mg, mL, or mm are each from the "ones" column.

INSTRUCTIONS TO CALCULATE MEDICATIONS BY WEIGHT

In some cases medications will be ordered based on the weight of the patient. Usually this requires the nurse to figure out what the patients weight is in kilograms (kg).

You may wish to practice this by taking your own weight in pounds, place it into your calculator and divide it by the conversion factor of 2.2.

The answer will be your weight in kg (might be nice to list this on your drivers license).

If the order reads: MedX 5mg/kg PO now you would read it "MedX 5 milligrams per (or for each) kilogram by mouth now"

STEPS:

1. Determine the patients weight in kilograms (Lbs divided by conversion factor 2.2)

2. Multiply the ordered medication by the number of kg.

3. Final answer is then what the physician really ordered.

Example:

Mr. James weighs 264 Lbs. The physician has ordered for MexX 5mg/kg as listed above.

1. 264 Lbs ÷ 2.2 = 120 kg

2. 5 mg • 120 kg = 600 mg

3. The physician really ordered **600 mg** to be given by mouth now to Mr. James.

Temperature Conversion

In the formulas below, / represents division, * represents multiplication, - subtraction, + addition and = is equal.

Tc = (5/9)*(Tf-32); Tc = temperature in degrees Celsius, Tf = temperature in degrees Fahrenheit

For example, suppose you have a Fahrenheit temperature of 98.6 degrees and you wanted to convert it into degrees on the Celsius scale. Using the above formula, you would first subtract 32 from the Fahrenheit temperature and get 66.6 as a result. Then you multiply 66.6 by five-ninths and get the converted value of 37 degrees Celsius.

Below is the formula to convert a Celsius scale temperature into degrees on the Fahrenheit scale.

Tf = (9/5)*Tc+32; Tc = temperature in degrees Celsius, Tf = temperature in degrees Fahrenheit

Assume that you have a Celsius scale temperature of 100 degrees and you wish to convert it into degrees on the Fahrenheit scale. Using the stated formula, you first multiply the Celsius scale temperature reading by nine-fifths and get a result of 180. Then add 32 to 180 and get the final converted result of 212 degrees on the Fahrenheit scale.

Below is another accepted conversion method that works just as well and perhaps might be easier to remember. No matter which direction you want to covert, Fahrenheit to Celsius or Celsius to Fahrenheit, always first add 40 to the number. Next, multiply by 5/9 or 9/5 just like the first method. Then, always subtract out the 40 you just added to yield the final result. To remember whether to use 5/9 or 9/5 when converting from Fahrenheit to Celsius or Celsius to Fahrenheit, just simply remember, F (for Fahrenheit) begins with the same letter as Fraction. 5/9 is always a Fraction; while 9/5 is also a fraction, in this form, it is Clearly a whole number plus a fraction (1 and 4/5). Thus, if you want to convert Fahrenheit (F) to Celsius (C), then use the Fraction 5/9; Celsius (C) to Fahrenheit (F), use the other, 9/5, which is Clearly not just a fraction.

For an example of this method, we'll use the values we used in the initial example, 98.6 F and 37 C, which are equal.

To convert from F to C, try these calculations manually.

98.6 + 40 = 138.6, and 138.6 * 5/9 = 77. For the final calculation, remove the 40. 77 - 40 = 37

To convert from C to F, try these calculations manually.

37 + 40 = 77, and 77 * 9/5 = 138.6. For the final calculation, remove the 40. 138.6 - 40 = 98.6

In summary, add 40, (F to C) multiply by Fraction...(C to F) multiply by the other, subtract 40.

The Celsius temperature scale is still sometimes referred to as the "centigrade" scale. Centigrade means "consisting of or divided into 100 degrees;" the Celsius scale, devised by Swedish Astronomer Andres Celsius (1701-1744) for scientific purposes, has 100 degrees between the freezing point (0 C) and boiling point (100 C) of pure water at sea level air pressure. The term Celsius was adopted in 1948 by an international conference on weights and measures.

Chapter 4 Sample QUIZ

Complete the following by using your Metric Conversion Chart, Step one of the Dosage Calculation Formula, or using the Ratio method of converting. Correct each problem prior to moving onto your next problem.

1. 100 Lbs = _____ KG

2. 155 Lbs = _____ KG

3. 180 Lbs = _____ KG

4. 2.5 g = _____ mg

5. 1500 mg = _____ g

6. 750 mg = _____ g

7. 0.5 g = _____ mg

8. 5 tsp = _____ mL

9. 2 Tbsp = _____ tsp

10. 5 mL's = _____ cc's

11. The surgical technologist is asked to maintain 60cc's of Marcaine on the back table for administration through the pain pump. How many ounce or ounce's is this equivalent to?

   a. 1   b. 2

   c. 3   c. 4

12. What is the ideal temperature range for the operating room in Celsius?

   a. 18°c to 22°c

   b. 28°c to 34°c

   c. 65°c to 72°c

   c. 10°c to 17°c

13. A patient enters the o.r. the chart reads the patient as weighing 180 lbs, the anesthesia provider ask you to read the chart and determine how many kilograms does the patient weighs?

   a. 47.34 kg

   b. 66.5 kg

   c. 81.81kg

   c. 100.1 kg

14. A surgeon asks you how many mL was used during the procedure. You look at your 20cc syringe and 15cc's were used during the case, what would be the correct response?

   a. 15mL

   b. 30mL

   c. 45mL

   d. 5mL

15. During a procedure a surgeon ask what is the amount of blood loss, you had started the procedure with 1L of .9% Sodium Chloride and the suction canister contains 500mL of fluids, you administered 3 60cc syringes of irrigation. Based on these figures how much blood loss had occurred?

   a. 1L

   b. 300mL

   c. 180mL

   c. 320mL

Chapter 4 Sample QUIZ ANSWERS

1. 45.45 KG

2. 70.45 KG

3. 81.81 KG

4. 2500 mg

5. 1.5 g

6. 0.75 g

7. 500 mg

8. 25 mL

9. 6 tsp

10. 5 cc's

11. (b) 2 ounces

12. (a) 18°c to 22°c= 65°f to 72°f

13. (c) 81.81

14. (a) 15mL cc and mL are equal

15. (d) 320mL the amount of irrigation used was 180cc=180ml, subtract 180mL from 500mL= 320m

Exam Preparation Tips

The Surgical Technologist Certification Exam is not the type of exam where you hope for a high test score by just studying the night before. Good study habits can have an impact on how well you do on the exam. **In order for you do perform well is to enter the exam relaxed and confident.**

Regular study time should be established. Each person studies best in different ways, but most importantly **you must pick a regular schedule to study.**

It's not how long you study but how comfortable you are with your surroundings while studying. **Eliminate any distractions that can disrupt your studies**, such as television, telephone, and even you family. Never lie down while studying; this will cause more exhaustion, and a tendency to sleep. Use a desk, a comfortable chair, and adequate light. If your home is too distracting then **go to the library or somewhere more conducive to study.**

It is important to get plenty of rest, and not skip meals. Your level of concentration during the exam can suffer if you lack proper nutrition. Coffee and other stimulants are not recommended.

1. Make sure you understand the meaning of every word you read.

2. Study uninterrupted for at least 30 minutes.

3. Simulate examinations conditions when studying.

4. Study alone, if possible, also form a study group to meet periodically.

5. Make sure you understand the answers to every question in this study guide.

6. Always follow the recommended technique for answering multiple-choice questions.

7. Always time yourself when doing practice questions.

8. Concentrate your study time in the areas of your greatest weakness.

9. Exercise regularly and stay in good physical condition.

10. Establish a schedule for studying and keep to it.

Test Taking Strategies

1. Read the directions; do not assume that you know what the directions are.

2. Be careful marking your answers;

    a. Mark only one answer for each question.
    b. Do not make extraneous markings on your answer sheet.
    c. Darken completely the allotted space for the answer you choose.
    d. Erase completely any answer that you change.

3. Be certain you are marking the proper answer.

4. Do not read into the question.

5. Always read the choices before you choose an answer.

6. Be aware of absolute words like **"never, none, nothing, nobody, always, all, everyone, everybody, only, and must"** are usually the wrong choice.

7. Transitional words such as **"and, also, and besides"** indicate there may be more than one part to the answer and both must be true to be correct.

8. Words like **"or, but, however"** show contrast and offer a choice of situations where only one part of the choice will be true.

9. Words like **"similarly, sometimes, generally, and possibly"** are comparison words and require you to make a judgment, leaving you more of choice to the correct answer.

10. Cross-out choices you know are wrong.

11. Be sure of the question before you answer it.

12. Never make a choice based on frequency of previous answers.

13. Only change an answer when you are positive it's wrong.

Oral Interview

You have succeeded in passing the Surgical Technologist Certification Exam some facilities require an oral interview with a clinical board, if this is the case, follow these recommended practices.

APPEARANCE

When appearing for oral interviews always dress appropriately. To make the best impression possible, you should consider the effect of clothes and grooming. The interviewers are trained to measure **skills** and not to be concerned with appearance. However, as human beings, they are still somewhat influenced by the ***first impression***.

It is best to come in a business suit. You should determine what colors suit you best to create a conservative but live appearance. This is the time to create a serious impression by ***dressing up***. Colors should be subdued. Dark blue and gray are always appropriate for business suit colors. For males a white, long sleeve shirt is the proper color for you interview, and the wearing of a tie is mandatory.

Attention should be paid to details such as clean fingernails and hair, polished shoes, and simple jewelry. Women should wear make-up and hairstyles that are businesslike and flattering. Avoid looking like you just walked out of a hair salon by getting your haircut well in advance. A business suit is recommended for ladies.

INTERVIEW TECHNIQUES

When entering the interview room **greet the interviewer** with a warm professional greeting, such as:

"Good afternoon sir (madam)." *Or* "Good afternoon"

Always reach out with your hand when greeting. **Do not sit until invited** to do so. If not invited to sit, ask in a professional manner

"May I?" (Pointing to the chair.)

When shaking hands with the interviewer make sure your handshake is firm and confident. Do not take control of the interviewers hand during the handshake; allow the interviewer to decide which style to choose from *"dominant"* (his/her hand above yours turning your palm up), *"submissive"* (his/her hand below with their palm facing up), or *"equals"* (his/her palm and your palm side by side).

The manner in which the interviewer shakes your hand sets the tone of the interview. If it's a *"dominate"* handshake he/she will lead the interview through questions and answers. With this type of interview answer questions in a manner that allows **him/her to be in control**.

An interviewer with a *"submissive"* handshake will allow **you to be in control** of the interview. **_This type of interview can be misleading._** You have to be cautious and not appear intimidating. Leave yourself a way out. Formulate your response in a manner in which the interviewer can respond. **Do not be definitive be open ended.**

An interviewer with a *"equals"* type handshake, will allow for the back and forth input. This too **must be approached with caution. You must know you place don't become complacent, you the one being interviewed.**

The interview should at all times be kept at a **professional level.** Avoid the pitfalls of common language. Do not respond in a manner that can be construed as degrading, or too familiar.

When responding to questions always think about the question first, and then about the response, then give your response. **Never be too quick to respond.** Occasionally place your hand to your chin, rubbing it gently as if you're in deep thought. This gives the appearance of a person who thinks before he/she acts displays a very positive trait.

When unsure of a question be sure to **ask the interviewer to repeat the question**, you don't want to answer a question that was not asked. Try not to repeat this action often.

At the conclusion of the interview, stand up and give your salutations to the interviewer such as: **"I would like to thank you for this opportunity, it was a pleasure meeting you, and I am looking forward to seeing you again."**

Reach out and extend your hand again. Turn and leave with confidence, **do not turn around** unless called upon. This gives the impression of confidence.

NOTE:

If there is more than one interviewer present utilize the same approach in a more generalized manner. *"I would like to thank you for this opportunity, it was a pleasure, and I am looking forward to seeing all of you again."*

A Practical Study Guide For The Surgical Technologist Certification Exam

MOCK CERTIFICATION EXAMINATION

PRACTICE EXAMINATION

DO NOT OPEN THE BOOK UNTIL READY TO BEGIN EXAM
CANDIDATE HAS 4 HOURS TO COMPLETE THIS EXAM
DO NOT WRITE IN THIS TEST BOOKLET

TEST BOOK 0001

NBSTA Mock Exam

Multiple Choice
Identify the choice that best completes the statement or answers the question.

1. Preoperative diagnostic studies are performed by the ____.
   a. medical laboratory
   b. diagnostic imaging department
   c. pathology department
   d. emergency department

2. The nonprofit organization that develops standards and performance criteria for health care organizations is the ____.
   a. Association of Perioperative Registered Nurses
   b. Association of Surgical Technologists
   c. American College of Surgeons
   d. The Joint Commission

3. *Accreditation* is a term that applies to ____.
   a. individuals
   b. programs
   c. program directors
   d. community colleges

4. A CRNA is part of which operating room group?
   a. anesthesia department
   b. sterile surgical team
   c. housekeeping department
   d. central supply department

5. A contractual relationship and mutual benefit that exist when one party or entity agrees to pay another for a specified loss or condition is known as ____.
   a. PPO
   b. insurance
   c. Medicare
   d. co-payment

6. Medicare is a program administered by the federal government through which agency?
   a. HCFA
   b. Social Security Administration
   c. Medicaid
   d. HMO

7. If an individual is concerned about an action that another individual is about to take, in what manner should the concern be handled?
   a. State the concern in the form of a question to the individual.
   b. Bring the concern to the attention of management.
   c. Fill out an incident report.
   d. Ask the person to leave the room.

8. Which term defines the relationship among the surgical technologist, the patient, and the patient's family?
   a. therapeutic
   b. professional
   c. social
   d. medical

9. A hospital that is owned by an individual or corporation in order to make a profit is known as which type of hospital?
   a. ambulatory
   b. charitable
   c. proprietary
   d. home based

10. What program allows for a surgical technologist to ascend to positions of increased responsibility?
    a. retention
    b. competency
    c. enhancement
    d. clinical ladder

11. Which department oversees the sterilization needs of the hospital?
    a. medical laboratory
    b. maintenance and biomed
    c. purchasing and central processing
    d. housekeeping

12. Which entity is responsible for verifying that the school attended by the surgical technologist meets national standards?
    a. NBSTSA
    b. CAAHEP
    c. ARC-ST
    d. AORN

13. Whose responsibility is it to identify the surgical patient?
    a. transportation personnel
    b. holding area nurse
    c. anesthesia provider
    d. all of the above

14. Who is responsible for checking diagnostic tests such as X-rays and CT scans to confirm the proper area or side before an incision is made?
    a. circulator
    b. surgeon
    c. anesthesia provider
    d. radiologist

15. What is used to report an unusual event that has occurred and may have legal ramifications for the staff or the patient?
    a. summary of action report
    b. incident report
    c. negligence report
    d. history of events report

16. The Patient's Bill of Rights establishes the patient as ____.
    a. dependent on health care providers
    b. the consumer of goods
    c. the secondary decision maker in care

d. having limited health care rights

17. Many professional codes have been incorporated into law and have some effect on judgments about professional conduct for litigation. Which of the following is not a professional code?
    a. AMA Principles of Medical Ethics
    b. AST Code of Ethics
    c. AORN Standards
    d. International Code of Nursing Ethics

18. Knowledge and skills required for the profession to provide effective and reliable services is called ____.
    a. competencies
    b. legal requirement
    c. policy
    d. scope of practice

19. To a very large extent, surgical technology and surgical assistant scope of practice is determined by the delegatory decisions made by the ____.
    a. supervising surgeon
    b. circulating nurse
    c. medical staff director
    d. hospital CEO

20. Which standard does the surgical technologist use as a guide in the establishment of entry-level knowledge and skills?
    a. AST code of ethics
    b. program accreditation standards
    c. Core Curriculum for Surgical Technologists
    d. continuing education guidelines

21. Who is responsible for ensuring accredited surgical technology programs are engaged in an ongoing quest for quality?
    a. ARC-ST
    b. NBSTSA
    c. CAAHEP
    d. AST

22. Hospitals are required to provide device manufacturers with information about patients with all EXCEPT ____.
    a. permanently implantable devices
    b. life-sustaining devices
    c. life-supporting devices
    d. incidents that reasonably suggest the probability that a medical device has caused or contributed to the death, serious injury, illness, or other adverse experience of a patient

23. To establish negligence, which of the following must be proven?
    a. The plaintiff must prove that the defendant had a duty to the plaintiff.
    b. The negligent conduct was not the cause of the harm to the plaintiff.
    c. The defendant departed from the standard of care.
    d. The defendant had the necessary education.

24. A uterine fibroid is an example of what type of factor causing surgical intervention?
    a. trauma
    b. genetic malformation
    c. nonmalignant neoplasm
    d. metabolic disease

25. All developmental theories must account for changes in which domain?
    a. financial
    b. philosophical
    c. cognitive
    d. ethical

26. One of the advantages to the life-stage approach is that it ____.
    a. focuses on sexual development
    b. explains cognitive development
    c. does not require advanced levels of education to apply
    d. explains affective learning

27. Any need or activity related to the identification and understanding of one's place in an organized universe (expressions may involve theology, philosophy, mythology, and intuition) is termed a ____ need.
    a. spiritual
    b. social
    c. physiological
    d. physical

28. What is the term given to a genetic malformation known commonly as a cleft lip?
    a. Conn's syndrome
    b. Cushing's syndrome
    c. crepitation
    d. cheiloschisis

29. Roy states that health involves becoming an integrated and ____ person.
    a. self-reliant
    b. whole
    c. accessible
    d. analytical

30. Which term describes the following coping mechanism: "A patient tries to give excuses as to why he or she has a particular illness"?
    a. regression
    b. rationalization
    c. denial
    d. repression

31. In which religion is organ donation controversial?
    a. Jewish
    b. Jehovah's Witness
    c. Buddhist
    d. Roman Catholic

32. Which of the following religions does not permit abortion under any circumstances?
    a. Jewish
    b. Protestant
    c. Buddhist
    d. Jehovah's Witness

33. A patient is considered a pediatric patient if he or she is between the ages of ____.
    a. 2 and 12
    b. birth and 10
    c. birth and 12
    d. 2 and 13

34. The term *neonate* applies to the pediatric patient who is between the ages of ____.
    a. birth and 14 days
    b. birth and 28 days
    c. 24 hours and 28 days
    d. 6 hours and 14 days

35. It is imperative that caregivers should deal with pediatric patients ____.
    a. quickly
    b. cautiously
    c. truthfully
    d. indifferently

36. Who should stand nearby to assist the anesthesia provider during induction of a pediatric patient?
    a. nurse's aide
    b. surgeon
    c. circulating surgical technologist
    d. STSR

37. If a pediatric patient has a pneumothorax, there is an accumulation of air in the ____.
    a. pleural cavity
    b. esophagus
    c. bronchial tree
    d. abdomen

38. Bleeding in a pediatric trauma patient must be controlled to prevent ____.
    a. brachial plexus injury
    b. infiltration
    c. distension
    d. severe hypovolemia

39. During birth, the most common bone fracture is of the ____.
    a. radius
    b. fibula
    c. clavicle
    d. skull

40. Which postoperative complication is not common for gastric bypass or gastroplasty surgery?
    a. suture rejection
    b. abdominal catastrophes
    c. internal hernia
    d. acute gastric distension

41. During abdominal procedures on patients who are obese, what procedure might additionally be performed due to newly identified pathology?
    a. pancreatectomy
    b. Whipple
    c. cholecystectomy
    d. splenectomy

42. Immediate operative intervention is performed on the pregnant patient for the following emergency procedures EXCEPT ____.
    a. appendicitis
    b. competent cervical os
    c. traumatic injury
    d. ectopic pregnancy

43. In the pregnant patient, what trimester is the ideal time to perform abdominal surgery?
    a. first
    b. second
    c. third
    d. not safe at anytime

44. What situation would present difficulties in the intubation of a patient with AIDS?
    a. dehydration
    b. hypovolemia
    c. Kaposi's sarcoma lesions
    d. pneumonia

45. The term *golden hour* refers to ____.
    a. terminally ill patients' last hours
    b. giving care to a trauma victim within an hour
    c. postoperative care
    d. controlling hemorrhage

46. The life-stage approach combines all of the following EXCEPT ____.
    a. social concerns
    b. physical concerns
    c. spiritual concerns
    d. environmental concerns

47. Tears are not produced until the age of ____ month(s).
    a. 0 to 1
    b. 2 to 3
    c. 1 to 2
    d. 3 to 4

48. For pediatric patients, ____ temperature is the primary means of monitoring temperature.
    a. oral
    b. esophageal
    c. rectal
    d. skin

49. Sulfonamides are associated with an increased incidence of ____.
    a. kernicterus
    b. gray syndrome
    c. torticollis
    d. electrolyte imbalance

50. In a patient who is post-gastric-bypass, respiratory failure often indicates ____.
    a. gaseous distention
    b. visceral perforation
    c. bowel strangulation
    d. peritonitis

51. When placing the pregnant surgical patient in the supine position, the circulating surgical technologist should place a small rolled pad or sheet under the right hip. This will help ____.
    a. take weight off of the vena cava
    b. make the patient more comfortable
    c. shift the uterus to gain better access to the abdominal contents
    d. prevent preterm labor

52. All of the following are clinical syndromes that require surgical intervention in the patient with AIDS EXCEPT ____.
    a. peritonitis
    b. pancreatitis
    c. non-Hodgkin's lymphoma
    d. mycobacterial infection of the retroperitoneum or spleen

53. Emergency procedures on geriatric patients are associated with ____.
    a. better preoperative planning
    b. higher mortality
    c. Trauma
    d. failure to minimize postoperative stress of hypothermia and hypoxemia

54. Three factors are important when considering the resulting injury that a patient will sustain from a trauma. These include ____.
    a. velocity, flexibility of tissue, and location of injury
    b. location of injury, shape of the injuring force, and velocity
    c. shape of the injuring force, flexibility of the tissue, and location of the injury
    d. velocity, flexibility of tissue, and shape of the injuring force

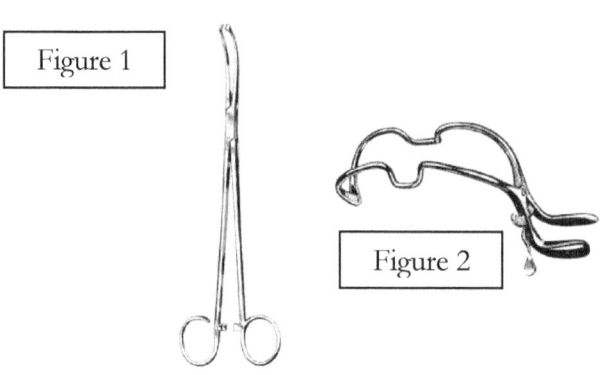
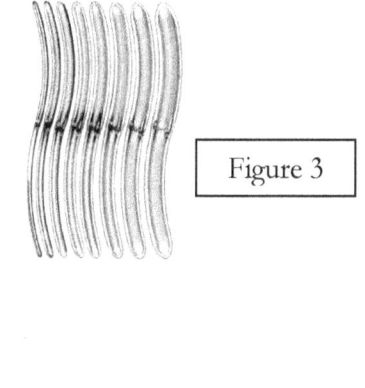

55. What is the name of the instrument displayed in figure 1?
    a. Allis
    b. Babcock
    c. White tonsil seizing forceps
    d. Schnidt tonsil forceps

56. What is the name of the instrument displayed in figure 2?
    a. Jennings mouth gag
    b. Wilson retractor
    c. Johnson tongue retractor
    d. Michigan clamp

57. What type of procedure would the instruments displayed in figure 3 used for?
    a. orthopedic
    b. general
    c. gyn
    d. neurological

58. What instruments would commonly be used in a tonsillectomy?
    a. 1 and 3
    b. 2 and 3
    c. 1 and 2
    d. 1, 2 and 3

59. The modem of a computer is a communication device that enables information to be sent over ____.
    a. telephone lines
    b. satellite systems
    c. cable networks
    d. television antennae

60. Materials that inhibit the flow of electrons are called ____.
    a. inhibitors
    b. insulators
    c. conductors
    d. refractors

61. The ____ coordinates operations of the computer.
    a. CPU
    b. hard drive
    c. Zip drive
    d. modem

62. A "hot wire" is usually identified as having ____.
    a. black-, white-, or red-colored insulation
    b. blue-, white-, or red-colored insulation
    c. white-, black-, or blue-colored insulation
    d. black-, blue-, or red-colored insulation

63. The active electrode is also called the ____.
    a. electrosurgical pencil
    b. grounding pad
    c. dispersive electrode
    d. inactive electrode

64. All are false regarding the grounding pad EXCEPT which of the following?
    a. The grounding pad is removed by the surgeon at the end of the procedure.
    b. A properly placed grounding pad can be the cause of severe patient burns.
    c. The grounding pad is used only when the ESU is operated in the monopolar mode.
    d. It is recommended to apply the grounding pad before the patient receives anesthesia.

65. Molecules carry thermal energy in the form of ____.
    a. motion
    b. passive energy
    c. a wave
    d. thermal equilibrium

66. Which term is used to describe "the multiplication of organisms in tissue"?
    a. nosocomial
    b. infection
    c. cross contamination
    d. culture

67. A nonliving particle that is completely reliant on the host cell for survival is called a ____.
    a. bacteria
    b. fungus
    c. protozoa
    d. virus

68. When stainless steel instruments are manually cleaned, a(n) ____ should be used to avoid scratching the surface of the instrument.
    a. circular motion
    b. abrasive cleanser
    c. wire brush
    d. back-and-forth motion

69. The ____ is used to remove small organic particles and soil from areas of instruments that are difficult to clean manually.
    a. ultrasonic washer
    b. CUSA
    c. wire brush
    d. gas sterilizer

70. Gas gangrene and cellulitis is caused by which microorganism?
    a. *Klebsiella pneumoniae*
    b. *Pasteurella multocida*
    c. *Clostridium perfringens*
    d. *E. coli*

71. An example of a pressure device that may be used to prevent deep-vein thrombosis is ____.
    a. a tourniquet
    b. a blood pressure cuff
    c. sequential stockings
    d. drains

72. When CPR must be accomplished through the sterile field, sterile team members should ____.
    a. stay sterile
    b. stand back and let the surgeon do the chest compressions
    c. do whatever procedures are necessary
    d. pay careful attention to the instruments and sharps

73. All are blood replacement products EXCEPT ____.
    a. whole blood
    b. plasma
    c. packed red blood cells
    d. vitamin K

74. Which type of drug name is advocated in the health care setting?
    a. chemical
    b. generic
    c. trade
    d. brand

75. Drug administered within a joint is ____.
    a. subcutaneous
    b. intravenous
    c. intra-articular
    d. dermal

76. Drugs with a high potential to cause psychological or physical dependence and abuse are called ____.
    a. over-the-counter medications
    b. chemical substances
    c. prescription medications
    d. controlled substances

77. Sellick's maneuver is also known as ____.
    a. cricoid pressure
    b. intubation
    c. tracheostomy
    d. ACLS

78. Which agents selectively interrupt the associative pathways of the brain?
    a. opioids
    b. dissociative
    c. induction
    d. tranquilizers

79. Which is the sole responsibility of the circulator?
    a. identify patient
    b. document physical findings
    c. document emotional status
    d. ensure preoperative duties completed

80. What drug is used to fight bacteria infections caused by anaerobic microbes?
    a. Flagyl
    b. Cefotan
    c. Ancef
    d. Cipro

81. Which anesthetic agent depresses the CNS when inhaled?
    a. nitrous oxide
    b. Demerol
    c. Halothane
    d. Mannitol

82. The generic name for Anectine is ____.
    a. curare
    b. papaverine
    c. succinylcholine
    d. bupivacaine

83. Which device is used to quickly deliver a large volume of blood or other fluid to the patient?
    a. Swan-Ganz catheter
    b. Bair Hugger
    c. rapid infusion pump
    d. spirometer

84. General abdominal procedures typically require a(n) ____ instrument set.
    a. ob-gyn
    b. laparotomy
    c. otorhinolaryngology
    d. peripheral vascular

85. Which of the following isolate and protect the operative site from contaminants?
    a. cuffs
    b. drapes
    c. tourniquets
    d. sponges

86. Sponges used for procedures requiring smaller incisions are called ____.
    a. laparotomy
    b. neurosurgical
    c. Raytec
    d. tonsil

87. The type of surgical dressing that eliminates dead space and prevents edema or postoperative bleeding is called ____.
    a. bulk
    b. pressure
    c. single-layer
    d. splint

88. A Minerva jacket ____.
    a. extends from the head to the hips
    b. is secured to the torso to support the hip or shoulder
    c. extends from the axillae to the hips
    d. extends from the neck to the mid-thigh region

89. The final wound classification is assigned when ____.
    a. an incision is made
    b. a wound is drained
    c. inflammation is present
    d. the procedure is finished

90. Which of the following sutures is absorbable?
    a. Dexon
    b. Mersilene
    c. tantalum
    d. silk

91. The area of tough connective tissue just beneath the skin and just above the subcutaneous layer is called ____.
    a. peritoneum
    b. fascia
    c. subcuticular
    d. muscle

92. Needles manufactured with suture strands inserted into one end are ____ needles.
    a. closed-eye
    b. French-eye
    c. swaged
    d. trocar

93. Needles used to penetrate tissue for the delivery of endoscopes into body cavities or joint spaces are ____ needles.
    a. conventional cutting
    b. reverse-cutting
    c. side-cutting
    d. trocar point

94. Another name given to "rapid-release" needles is ____.
    a. quick close
    b. endoclose
    c. control-release
    d. quick tie

95. The sterile field should be established ____.
    a. close to the door
    b. in the middle of the room
    c. farthest from the door
    d. in major traffic paths

96. Which of the following provides a large, sterile area for initial preparation and storage of drapes, supplies, irrigations, medicines, and instruments?
    a. operating room table
    b. back table
    c. prep stand
    d. Mayo stand

97. Which instrument(s) are placed pencil style into the surgeon's hand?
    a. sponges
    b. ringed instruments
    c. scalpel
    d. needle holders

98. When changing into operating room attire, the _____ must be donned first.
    a. scrub shirt
    b. hair cover
    c. scrub pants
    d. shoe covers

99. Which statement is true regarding recommendations for double gloving?
    a. Fat is known to degrade latex.
    b. The barrier efficiency of latex increases over time.
    c. Studies show that visible contamination of the hands occurred in 50% of the cases with single gloving.
    d. Extra comfort may be achieved by wearing an under glove of the normal size and an outer glove one-half size larger.

100. Which statement is true regarding urinary catheterization?
    a. The balloon is inflated with saline.
    b. The circulator will determine the size and style of the catheter.
    c. Use the largest size that will drain the bladder and prevent leakage.
    d. If used to inflate the balloon, air may escape and cause an embolism.

101. Thoracentesis is the removal of _____.
    a. CSF for laboratory analysis
    b. fluid from the pleural cavity
    c. fluid from the peritoneal cavity
    d. fluid from a joint space

102. An estimation of the arterial levels of carbon dioxide is determined with the use of _____.
    a. pulse oximetry
    b. capnography
    c. arterial blood gases
    d. plethysmography

103. The normal range for the hemoglobin of a female is _____.
    a. 40% to 52%
    b. 35% to 46%
    c. 13.5% to 18%
    d. 11.5% to 15.5%

104. For which purpose does a surgeon use a suture on a specimen?
    a. to hold the tissue together
    b. to identify margins
    c. to allow for easy handoff to the circulator
    d. the preferred method of pathologists

105. Nissen fundoplication is the procedure performed to correct a(n) _____.
    a. gastric ulcer
    b. inguinal hernia
    c. hiatal hernia
    d. ruptured tubal pregnancy

106. Segmental resection of the breast refers to the removal of
    a. only the tumor
    b. a portion of the tumor for biopsy
    c. the tumor and a reasonable margin of healthy tissue
    d. the entire breast and axillary nodes

107. Mastectomy is the removal of the _____.
    a. entire mammary breast
    b. entire breast and pectoral muscles
    c. entire breast, pectoral muscles, and axillary lymph nodes
    d. tumor only, preserving subcutaneous tissue for reconstruction

108. Which hormone increases the calcium levels in the blood?
    a. calcitonin
    b. parathyroid
    c. thyroxine
    d. thymosin

109. Complications of thyrotoxicosis include _____.
    a. hoarseness
    b. thyroid storm
    c. skeletal damage
    d. esophageal compression

110. The ligament that supports the bulk of the ovary is called the _____ ligament.
    a. broad
    b. round
    c. suspensory
    d. cardinal

111. The uterine appendages are the _____.
    a. appendix and fallopian tubes
    b. fallopian tubes and the salpinx
    c. ovaries and the appendix
    d. ovaries and fallopian tubes

112. In which position is the patient generally placed into for a D and C?
    a. frog-leg
    b. sitting
    c. lithotomy
    d. Trendelenburg

113. The perineum in the female is the area between which two structures?
    a. vaginal opening and anus
    b. labia majora and labia minora
    c. clitoris and labia minora
    d. urethral meatus and vestibule

114. What is another name given to an anterior and posterior repair?
    a. chondroplasty
    b. cystoplasty
    c. cystorrhaphy
    d. colporrhaphy

115. The innermost tunic of the eye is the ____.
    a. retina
    b. sclera
    c. choroid
    d. ciliary body

116. What is the action of acetylcholine chloride?
    a. to dilate the pupil
    b. to constrict the pupil
    c. to lower IOP
    d. to soften the zonules

117. Vitrectomy requires the use of what piece of specialized equipment?
    a. phacoemulsification unit
    b. cryotherapy unit
    c. diathermy unit
    d. ocutome

118. Mydriatics and cycloplegic drugs cause ____.
    a. pupil constriction
    b. shrinkage of the vitreous body
    c. reduction in inflammation
    d. pupil dilation

119. Enucleation is indicated for all EXCEPT ____.
    a. malignant neoplasm
    b. penetrating wounds
    c. extensive damage to vision
    d. intraocular pressure

120. Hemorrhage from the nose is described as ____.
    a. rhinorrhea
    b. sinusitis
    c. epistaxis
    d. hypertrophy

121. What is the name of the procedure that is used to change the external appearance of the nose?
    a. septoplasty
    b. submucous resection
    c. rhinoplasty
    d. intranasal antrostomy

122. During a tonsillectomy, which instrument can be used to put tension on the tonsil during dissection?
    a. Jensen Middleton
    b. long Allis
    c. Rosen knife
    d. Aufricht retractor

123. Coral is a type of _____.
    a. xenograft
    b. autograft
    c. homograft
    d. synthetic graft

124. What type of incision is made at the patient's hairline and can be bilaterally extended?
    a. coronal
    b. circular calvarial
    c. supraorbital
    d. intraoral

125. Endoscopic viewing of a joint is called _____.
    a. arthroplasty
    b. arthrotomy
    c. arthroscopy
    d. arthrocentesis

126. What surgical procedure is performed to remove hypertrophic breast tissue?
    a. augmentation mammoplasty
    b. reduction mammoplasty
    c. reconstructive mammoplasty
    d. mastectomy

127. Which instrument is NOT typically found in a plastic surgery instrument set?
    a. Berry needle holders
    b. Castroviejo needle holders
    c. iris scissors
    d. jeweler's forceps

128. All of the following are true for liposuction EXCEPT that it _____.
    a. can be used for body contouring
    b. can be used as a permanent means of weight loss
    c. can be performed on almost any area of the body
    d. is performed under general anesthesia

129. Which layer of epidermis is found only in the thick skin areas such as the palms of the hands and soles of the feet?
    a. stratum basale
    b. stratum lucidum
    c. stratum corneum
    d. stratum granulosum

130. A freely movable joint is known as which type of joint?
    a. hemarthrosis
    b. ampiarthrosis
    c. synarthrosis
    d. diarthrosis

131. All of the following are false for prostatectomy EXCEPT that _____.
    a. retropubic prostatectomy involves incising the bladder
    b. suprapubic prostatectomy involves a prostatic capsulotomy
    c. perineal prostatectomy provides good exposure to the fossa
    d. transurethral prostatectomy has increased incidence of postoperative infection

132. What do the medulla of the adrenal glands secrete?
    a. steroid hormones
    b. norepinephrine
    c. mineralocorticoids
    d. FSH

133. The condition of undescended testes is called _____.
    a. cryptorchidism
    b. testicular torsion
    c. hypospadias
    d. ESRD

134. Extending the foot at the ankle is referred to as _____.
    a. abduction
    b. dorsiflexion
    c. plantar flexion
    d. pronation

135. Which hemostatic agent is NOT used in orthopedics?
    a. Gelfoam
    b. bone wax
    c. thrombin
    d. oxidized cellulose

136. How many components are implanted during a total knee arthroplasty?
    a. one
    b. two
    c. three
    d. four

137. The concave indentation that serves as the socket for the head of the femur is the _____.
    a. glenoid
    b. acetabulum
    c. greater trochanter
    d. ilium

138. This chemical is also referred to as bone cement.
    a. methyl methacrylate
    b. ketorolac tromethamine
    c. cephalexin monohydrate
    d. phenylephrine hydrochloride

139. What two bones are involved in a patella tendon harvest for an ACL reconstruction?
    a. tibia, femur
    b. patella, femur
    c. tibia, patella
    d. fibula, tibia

140. Which artery supplies blood to the walls of the left atrium and ventricle?
    a. left anterior descending
    b. left main
    c. circumflex
    d. marginal

141. Which structure is attached to the valvular cusps and prevents valves from swinging back into the atria?
    a. papillary muscle
    b. myocardium
    c. chordae tendineae
    d. Purkinje fibers

142. The microscopic air sacs clustered at the end of the bronchiole are the ____.
    a. alveolar ducts
    b. alveoli
    c. alveolar pores
    d. bronchioles

143. Which of the following defines the term *systole*?
    a. no heartbeat
    b. contraction phase
    c. relaxation phase
    d. fibrillation

144. All of the following are false for aortic cannulation during cardiopulmonary bypass EXCEPT that the cannula is placed in the ____.
    a. right atrium
    b. aorta
    c. left ventricle
    d. subclavian artery

145. What is the number of true ribs?
    a. 2
    b. 3
    c. 7
    d. 12

146. Which is the most common complaint in the patient with a thoracic aorta aneurysm?
    a. tachycardia
    b. chest pain
    c. bradycardia
    d. dyspnea

147. Which study is best for determining the overall size of the heart and great vessel configuration?
    a. CT scan
    b. MRI
    c. AP and lateral X-rays
    d. electrocardiography

148. The surgical excision of a dilated portion of the aortic wall with immediate reconstruction using a synthetic graft is known as an ____.
    a. abdominal aortic aneurysm resection
    b. abdominal aortic aneurysm recession
    c. aortofemoral bypass
    d. aortopopliteal bypass

149. The primary purpose of a femoral-popliteal bypass is to ____.
    a. excise an aneurysm and reconstruct with a synthetic graft
    b. restore blood flow to the lower limb
    c. eliminate excess plaque from the femoral artery
    d. remove an atheroma from the popliteal vein

150. A Fogarty balloon catheter is used for a(n) ____.
    a. arterial embolectomy
    b. arteriovenous shunt
    c. carotid endarterectomy
    d. femoral-popliteal bypass

151. Which vein drains the deep veins of the foot?
    a. tibial artery
    b. tibial vein
    c. popliteal artery
    d. popliteal vein

152. A congenital collection of abnormal vessels of the brain that increase in size with time best describes a(n) ____.
    a. arteriovenous malformation
    b. cerebral aneurysm
    c. epidural hematoma
    d. subdural hematoma

153. Which system is responsible for distinguishing between favorable or unfavorable outside stimuli?
    a. amygdaloid
    b. limbic
    c. Monro
    d. Wernicke's

154. The midbrain is located between the ____.
    a. diencephalon and pons
    b. cerebrum and diencephalon
    c. medulla oblongata and midbrain
    d. mesencephalon and pons

155. What nerve controls the voluntary muscles of the pharynx, larynx, palate, sternocleidomastoid, and trapezius?
    a. accessory
    b. hypoglossal
    c. glossopharyngeal
    d. abducens

A 50 year old female enters the emergency department complaining of Dysmenorrhea and Menorrhagia, after examination and ultrasound, the attending physician notifies the charge nurse to schedule the patient for surgery.

Using the above scenario answer questions 156-160

156. As the surgical technologist what type of procedure should you anticipate to prepare for?
    a. Abdominal Procedure
    b. Genitourniary Procedure
    c. Gynecological Procedure
    d. Both a and c

157. As the surgical technologist what instrumentation should be pulled for the procedure?
    a. Gynecological Tray
    b. Hysterectomy Tray
    c. D and C Tray
    d. Both a and b

158. What equipment should be made available in the operating room suite?
    a. Electrocautery, Stirups, Video Tower
    b. Stirups, Suction, Video Tower
    c. Electrocautery, Stirups, Suction
    d. Suction, Video Tower, Laser Unit

159. What type of supplies would be pulled for this procedure?
    a. Laparotomy Custom Pack
    b. Spinal Custom Pack
    c. OB/GYN Custom Pack
    d. Hysterscopy Custom Pack

160. After analyzing the information what is the highest probability the procedure to be performed will be?
    a. Appendectomy
    b. Hysterectomy
    c. Cholecystectomy
    d. Colon Resection

A 40 year old male patient enters the emergency department exhibiting the following symptoms:
  Jaundice
  Right Upper Quadrant Pain
  Elevated White Blood Count

Using the above scenario answer questions 161-165

161. What would the most common cause of these symptoms?
    a. cholelithiasis
    b. inguinal hernia
    c. appendicitis
    d. obstructed colon

162. What is the function of a T-tube?
    a. drain urine
    b. drain chime
    c. drain bile
    d. drain blood

163. What position is used to displace the abdominal contents to enhance the surgeon's view of the lower abdominal region?
    a. Trendelenburg
    b. lateral
    c. Fowler's
    d. reverse Trendelenburg

164. In addition to a major general surgical instrumentation set, which of the following will also be needed for a cholecystectomy?
    a. rib resection instruments
    b. thoracic instruments
    c. CBD exploration instruments
    d. genitourinary instruments

165. Removal of the gallbladder is called ____.
    a. cholecystectomy
    b. choledochojejunostomy
    c. cholelithiasis
    d. colectomy

166. Which of the following instrument sets is this instrument located?
    a. Neurosurgical
    b. Plastic
    c. Tracheal
    d. Orthopedic

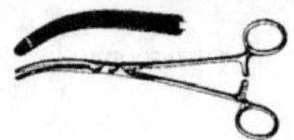

167. Which of the following instrument sets is this instrument located?
    a. Gall Bladder
    b. Plastic
    c. Ob-Gyn
    d. Genitourinary

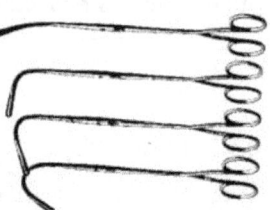

168. The name of this instrument is a/an
    a. Guyon vessel clamp
    b. Randall kidney stone forcep
    c. Herrick kidney pedicle clamp
    d. Wertheim pedicle clamp

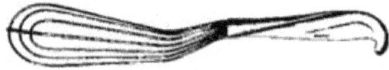

169. The name of this retractor is a/an
    a. Harrington
    b. Finochietto
    c. Davidson
    d. Allison

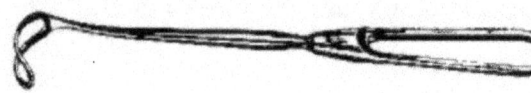

170. The name of this retractor is the
    a. Green thyroid
    b. Senn
    c. Hohmann
    d. Cushing

171. The name of this osteotome is a/an
    a. Hibbs
    b. Hoke
    c. Lambotte
    d. Smith-Petersen

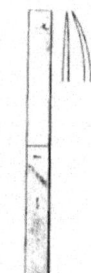

172. The name of this scissor is a/an
    a. Iris
    b. Potts-Smith
    c. Jorgenson
    d. Cottle

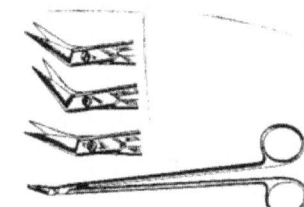

173. Which of the following instrument sets is this instrument located?
    a. Genitourinary
    b. Neurosurgical
    c. Orthopedic
    d. Cardiovascular

174. The name of this forceps is a/an
    a. DeBakey
    b. Adson
    c. Bonney
    d. Gerald

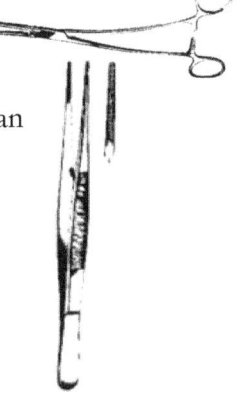

175. Identify the instrument shown on right
    a. Addson-Brown tissue forceps
    b. Addson-Beckman tissue forceps
    c. Russian tissue forceps
    d. DeBakey tissue forceps

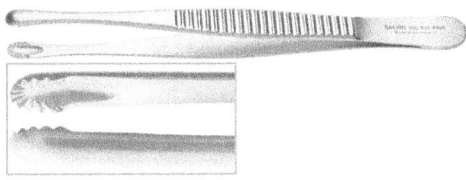

THIS PAGE IS INTENTIONALY LEFT BLANK

NBSTA Mock Exam

NAME: _____ DATE: _____ EXAM NUMBER___

MULTIPLE CHOICE

1. Ⓐ Ⓑ Ⓒ Ⓓ Ⓔ
2. Ⓐ Ⓑ Ⓒ Ⓓ Ⓔ
3. Ⓐ Ⓑ Ⓒ Ⓓ Ⓔ
4. Ⓐ Ⓑ Ⓒ Ⓓ Ⓔ
5. Ⓐ Ⓑ Ⓒ Ⓓ Ⓔ
6. Ⓐ Ⓑ Ⓒ Ⓓ Ⓔ
7. Ⓐ Ⓑ Ⓒ Ⓓ Ⓔ
8. Ⓐ Ⓑ Ⓒ Ⓓ Ⓔ
9. Ⓐ Ⓑ Ⓒ Ⓓ Ⓔ
10. Ⓐ Ⓑ Ⓒ Ⓓ Ⓔ
11. Ⓐ Ⓑ Ⓒ Ⓓ Ⓔ
12. Ⓐ Ⓑ Ⓒ Ⓓ Ⓔ
13. Ⓐ Ⓑ Ⓒ Ⓓ Ⓔ
14. Ⓐ Ⓑ Ⓒ Ⓓ Ⓔ
15. Ⓐ Ⓑ Ⓒ Ⓓ Ⓔ
16. Ⓐ Ⓑ Ⓒ Ⓓ Ⓔ
17. Ⓐ Ⓑ Ⓒ Ⓓ Ⓔ
18. Ⓐ Ⓑ Ⓒ Ⓓ Ⓔ
19. Ⓐ Ⓑ Ⓒ Ⓓ Ⓔ
20. Ⓐ Ⓑ Ⓒ Ⓓ Ⓔ
21. Ⓐ Ⓑ Ⓒ Ⓓ Ⓔ
22. Ⓐ Ⓑ Ⓒ Ⓓ Ⓔ
23. Ⓐ Ⓑ Ⓒ Ⓓ Ⓔ
24. Ⓐ Ⓑ Ⓒ Ⓓ Ⓔ
25. Ⓐ Ⓑ Ⓒ Ⓓ Ⓔ
26. Ⓐ Ⓑ Ⓒ Ⓓ Ⓔ
27. Ⓐ Ⓑ Ⓒ Ⓓ Ⓔ
28. Ⓐ Ⓑ Ⓒ Ⓓ Ⓔ
29. Ⓐ Ⓑ Ⓒ Ⓓ Ⓔ
30. Ⓐ Ⓑ Ⓒ Ⓓ Ⓔ
31. Ⓐ Ⓑ Ⓒ Ⓓ Ⓔ
32. Ⓐ Ⓑ Ⓒ Ⓓ Ⓔ
33. Ⓐ Ⓑ Ⓒ Ⓓ Ⓔ
34. Ⓐ Ⓑ Ⓒ Ⓓ Ⓔ
35. Ⓐ Ⓑ Ⓒ Ⓓ Ⓔ
36. Ⓐ Ⓑ Ⓒ Ⓓ Ⓔ
37. Ⓐ Ⓑ Ⓒ Ⓓ Ⓔ
38. Ⓐ Ⓑ Ⓒ Ⓓ Ⓔ
39. Ⓐ Ⓑ Ⓒ Ⓓ Ⓔ
40. Ⓐ Ⓑ Ⓒ Ⓓ Ⓔ
41. Ⓐ Ⓑ Ⓒ Ⓓ Ⓔ
42. Ⓐ Ⓑ Ⓒ Ⓓ Ⓔ
43. Ⓐ Ⓑ Ⓒ Ⓓ Ⓔ
44. Ⓐ Ⓑ Ⓒ Ⓓ Ⓔ
45. Ⓐ Ⓑ Ⓒ Ⓓ Ⓔ
46. Ⓐ Ⓑ Ⓒ Ⓓ Ⓔ
47. Ⓐ Ⓑ Ⓒ Ⓓ Ⓔ
48. Ⓐ Ⓑ Ⓒ Ⓓ Ⓔ
49. Ⓐ Ⓑ Ⓒ Ⓓ Ⓔ
50. Ⓐ Ⓑ Ⓒ Ⓓ Ⓔ
51. Ⓐ Ⓑ Ⓒ Ⓓ Ⓔ
52. Ⓐ Ⓑ Ⓒ Ⓓ Ⓔ
53. Ⓐ Ⓑ Ⓒ Ⓓ Ⓔ
54. Ⓐ Ⓑ Ⓒ Ⓓ Ⓔ
55. Ⓐ Ⓑ Ⓒ Ⓓ Ⓔ
56. Ⓐ Ⓑ Ⓒ Ⓓ Ⓔ
57. Ⓐ Ⓑ Ⓒ Ⓓ Ⓔ
58. Ⓐ Ⓑ Ⓒ Ⓓ Ⓔ
59. Ⓐ Ⓑ Ⓒ Ⓓ Ⓔ
60. Ⓐ Ⓑ Ⓒ Ⓓ Ⓔ
61. Ⓐ Ⓑ Ⓒ Ⓓ Ⓔ
62. Ⓐ Ⓑ Ⓒ Ⓓ Ⓔ
63. Ⓐ Ⓑ Ⓒ Ⓓ Ⓔ
64. Ⓐ Ⓑ Ⓒ Ⓓ Ⓔ
65. Ⓐ Ⓑ Ⓒ Ⓓ Ⓔ
66. Ⓐ Ⓑ Ⓒ Ⓓ Ⓔ
67. Ⓐ Ⓑ Ⓒ Ⓓ Ⓔ
68. Ⓐ Ⓑ Ⓒ Ⓓ Ⓔ
69. Ⓐ Ⓑ Ⓒ Ⓓ Ⓔ
70. Ⓐ Ⓑ Ⓒ Ⓓ Ⓔ
71. Ⓐ Ⓑ Ⓒ Ⓓ Ⓔ
72. Ⓐ Ⓑ Ⓒ Ⓓ Ⓔ
73. Ⓐ Ⓑ Ⓒ Ⓓ Ⓔ
74. Ⓐ Ⓑ Ⓒ Ⓓ Ⓔ
75. Ⓐ Ⓑ Ⓒ Ⓓ Ⓔ
76. Ⓐ Ⓑ Ⓒ Ⓓ Ⓔ
77. Ⓐ Ⓑ Ⓒ Ⓓ Ⓔ
78. Ⓐ Ⓑ Ⓒ Ⓓ Ⓔ
79. Ⓐ Ⓑ Ⓒ Ⓓ Ⓔ
80. Ⓐ Ⓑ Ⓒ Ⓓ Ⓔ
81. Ⓐ Ⓑ Ⓒ Ⓓ Ⓔ
82. Ⓐ Ⓑ Ⓒ Ⓓ Ⓔ
83. Ⓐ Ⓑ Ⓒ Ⓓ Ⓔ
84. Ⓐ Ⓑ Ⓒ Ⓓ Ⓔ
85. Ⓐ Ⓑ Ⓒ Ⓓ Ⓔ
86. Ⓐ Ⓑ Ⓒ Ⓓ Ⓔ
87. Ⓐ Ⓑ Ⓒ Ⓓ Ⓔ
88. Ⓐ Ⓑ Ⓒ Ⓓ Ⓔ
89. Ⓐ Ⓑ Ⓒ Ⓓ Ⓔ
90. Ⓐ Ⓑ Ⓒ Ⓓ Ⓔ
91. Ⓐ Ⓑ Ⓒ Ⓓ Ⓔ
92. Ⓐ Ⓑ Ⓒ Ⓓ Ⓔ
93. Ⓐ Ⓑ Ⓒ Ⓓ Ⓔ
94. Ⓐ Ⓑ Ⓒ Ⓓ Ⓔ
95. Ⓐ Ⓑ Ⓒ Ⓓ Ⓔ
96. Ⓐ Ⓑ Ⓒ Ⓓ Ⓔ
97. Ⓐ Ⓑ Ⓒ Ⓓ Ⓔ
98. Ⓐ Ⓑ Ⓒ Ⓓ Ⓔ
99. Ⓐ Ⓑ Ⓒ Ⓓ Ⓔ
100. Ⓐ Ⓑ Ⓒ Ⓓ Ⓔ
101. Ⓐ Ⓑ Ⓒ Ⓓ Ⓔ
102. Ⓐ Ⓑ Ⓒ Ⓓ Ⓔ
103. Ⓐ Ⓑ Ⓒ Ⓓ Ⓔ
104. Ⓐ Ⓑ Ⓒ Ⓓ Ⓔ
105. Ⓐ Ⓑ Ⓒ Ⓓ Ⓔ
106. Ⓐ Ⓑ Ⓒ Ⓓ Ⓔ
107. Ⓐ Ⓑ Ⓒ Ⓓ Ⓔ
108. Ⓐ Ⓑ Ⓒ Ⓓ Ⓔ
109. Ⓐ Ⓑ Ⓒ Ⓓ Ⓔ
110. Ⓐ Ⓑ Ⓒ Ⓓ Ⓔ
111. Ⓐ Ⓑ Ⓒ Ⓓ Ⓔ
112. Ⓐ Ⓑ Ⓒ Ⓓ Ⓔ
113. Ⓐ Ⓑ Ⓒ Ⓓ Ⓔ
114. Ⓐ Ⓑ Ⓒ Ⓓ Ⓔ
115. Ⓐ Ⓑ Ⓒ Ⓓ Ⓔ
116. Ⓐ Ⓑ Ⓒ Ⓓ Ⓔ
117. Ⓐ Ⓑ Ⓒ Ⓓ Ⓔ
118. Ⓐ Ⓑ Ⓒ Ⓓ Ⓔ
119. Ⓐ Ⓑ Ⓒ Ⓓ Ⓔ
120. Ⓐ Ⓑ Ⓒ Ⓓ Ⓔ
121. Ⓐ Ⓑ Ⓒ Ⓓ Ⓔ
122. Ⓐ Ⓑ Ⓒ Ⓓ Ⓔ
123. Ⓐ Ⓑ Ⓒ Ⓓ Ⓔ
124. Ⓐ Ⓑ Ⓒ Ⓓ Ⓔ
125. Ⓐ Ⓑ Ⓒ Ⓓ Ⓔ
126. Ⓐ Ⓑ Ⓒ Ⓓ Ⓔ
127. Ⓐ Ⓑ Ⓒ Ⓓ Ⓔ
128. Ⓐ Ⓑ Ⓒ Ⓓ Ⓔ
129. Ⓐ Ⓑ Ⓒ Ⓓ Ⓔ
130. Ⓐ Ⓑ Ⓒ Ⓓ Ⓔ
131. Ⓐ Ⓑ Ⓒ Ⓓ Ⓔ
132. Ⓐ Ⓑ Ⓒ Ⓓ Ⓔ
133. Ⓐ Ⓑ Ⓒ Ⓓ Ⓔ
134. Ⓐ Ⓑ Ⓒ Ⓓ Ⓔ
135. Ⓐ Ⓑ Ⓒ Ⓓ Ⓔ
136. Ⓐ Ⓑ Ⓒ Ⓓ Ⓔ
137. Ⓐ Ⓑ Ⓒ Ⓓ Ⓔ
138. Ⓐ Ⓑ Ⓒ Ⓓ Ⓔ
139. Ⓐ Ⓑ Ⓒ Ⓓ Ⓔ
140. Ⓐ Ⓑ Ⓒ Ⓓ Ⓔ
141. Ⓐ Ⓑ Ⓒ Ⓓ Ⓔ
142. Ⓐ Ⓑ Ⓒ Ⓓ Ⓔ
143. Ⓐ Ⓑ Ⓒ Ⓓ Ⓔ
144. Ⓐ Ⓑ Ⓒ Ⓓ Ⓔ
145. Ⓐ Ⓑ Ⓒ Ⓓ Ⓔ
146. Ⓐ Ⓑ Ⓒ Ⓓ Ⓔ
147. Ⓐ Ⓑ Ⓒ Ⓓ Ⓔ
148. Ⓐ Ⓑ Ⓒ Ⓓ Ⓔ
149. Ⓐ Ⓑ Ⓒ Ⓓ Ⓔ
150. Ⓐ Ⓑ Ⓒ Ⓓ Ⓔ
151. Ⓐ Ⓑ Ⓒ Ⓓ Ⓔ
152. Ⓐ Ⓑ Ⓒ Ⓓ Ⓔ
153. Ⓐ Ⓑ Ⓒ Ⓓ Ⓔ
154. Ⓐ Ⓑ Ⓒ Ⓓ Ⓔ
155. Ⓐ Ⓑ Ⓒ Ⓓ Ⓔ
156. Ⓐ Ⓑ Ⓒ Ⓓ Ⓔ
157. Ⓐ Ⓑ Ⓒ Ⓓ Ⓔ
158. Ⓐ Ⓑ Ⓒ Ⓓ Ⓔ
159. Ⓐ Ⓑ Ⓒ Ⓓ Ⓔ
160. Ⓐ Ⓑ Ⓒ Ⓓ Ⓔ
161. Ⓐ Ⓑ Ⓒ Ⓓ Ⓔ
162. Ⓐ Ⓑ Ⓒ Ⓓ Ⓔ
163. Ⓐ Ⓑ Ⓒ Ⓓ Ⓔ
164. Ⓐ Ⓑ Ⓒ Ⓓ Ⓔ
165. Ⓐ Ⓑ Ⓒ Ⓓ Ⓔ
166. Ⓐ Ⓑ Ⓒ Ⓓ Ⓔ
167. Ⓐ Ⓑ Ⓒ Ⓓ Ⓔ
168. Ⓐ Ⓑ Ⓒ Ⓓ Ⓔ
169. Ⓐ Ⓑ Ⓒ Ⓓ Ⓔ
170. Ⓐ Ⓑ Ⓒ Ⓓ Ⓔ
171. Ⓐ Ⓑ Ⓒ Ⓓ Ⓔ
172. Ⓐ Ⓑ Ⓒ Ⓓ Ⓔ
173. Ⓐ Ⓑ Ⓒ Ⓓ Ⓔ
174. Ⓐ Ⓑ Ⓒ Ⓓ Ⓔ
175. Ⓐ Ⓑ Ⓒ Ⓓ Ⓔ

NBSTA Mock Exam
NBSTA Mock Exam Test 1
Answer Section
MULTIPLE CHOICE

1. ANS: B
2. ANS: D
3. ANS: B
4. ANS: A
5. ANS: B
6. ANS: A
7. ANS: A
8. ANS: A
9. ANS: C
10. ANS: D
11. ANS: C
12. ANS: C
13. ANS: D
14. ANS: B
15. ANS: B
16. ANS: B
17. ANS: C
18. ANS: D
19. ANS: A
20. ANS: C
21. ANS: A
22. ANS: D
23. ANS: A
24. ANS: C
25. ANS: C
26. ANS: C
27. ANS: A
28. ANS: D
29. ANS: B
30. ANS: B
31. ANS: C
32. ANS: D
33. ANS: C
34. ANS: B
35. ANS: C
36. ANS: C
37. ANS: A
38. ANS: D
39. ANS: C
40. ANS: A
41. ANS: C
42. ANS: B
43. ANS: B
44. ANS: C
45. ANS: B
46. ANS: D
47. ANS: B
48. ANS: D
49. ANS: A
50. ANS: D
51. ANS: A
52. ANS: B
53. ANS: B
54. ANS: D
55. ANS: C
56. ANS: A
57. ANS: C
58. ANS: C
59. ANS: A
60. ANS: B
61. ANS: A
62. ANS: D
63. ANS: A
64. ANS: C
65. ANS: A
66. ANS: B
67. ANS: D
68. ANS: D
69. ANS: A
70. ANS: C
71. ANS: C
72. ANS: C
73. ANS: D
74. ANS: B
75. ANS: C
76. ANS: D
77. ANS: A
78. ANS: B
79. ANS: D
80. ANS: A
81. ANS: C
82. ANS: C
83. ANS: C
84. ANS: B
85. ANS: B
86. ANS: C
87. ANS: B
88. ANS: A
89. ANS: D
90. ANS: A
91. ANS: C
92. ANS: C
93. ANS: D
94. ANS: C
95. ANS: C
96. ANS: B
97. ANS: C
98. ANS: B
99. ANS: A
100. ANS: D
101. ANS: B
102. ANS: B
103. ANS: D
104. ANS: C
105. ANS: C
106. ANS: C
107. ANS: A
108. ANS: B
109. ANS: B
110. ANS: C
111. ANS: D
112. ANS: C
113. ANS: A
114. ANS: D
115. ANS: A
116. ANS: B
117. ANS: D
118. ANS: D
119. ANS: D
120. ANS: C
121. ANS: C
122. ANS: B
123. ANS: A
124. ANS: A
125. ANS: C
126. ANS: B
127. ANS: A
128. ANS: B
129. ANS: B
130. ANS: D
131. ANS: C
132. ANS: B
133. ANS: A
134. ANS: C
135. ANS: D
136. ANS: D
137. ANS: B
138. ANS: A
139. ANS: C
140. ANS: C
141. ANS: C
142. ANS: B
143. ANS: B
144. ANS: B
145. ANS: C
146. ANS: B
147. ANS: C
148. ANS: A
149. ANS: B
150. ANS: A
151. ANS: B
152. ANS: A
153. ANS: B
154. ANS: A
155. ANS: A
156. ANS: D
157. ANS: D
158. ANS: C
159. ANS: A
160. ANS: B
161. ANS: A
162. ANS: C
163. ANS: A
164. ANS: C
165. ANS: A
166. ANS: D
167. ANS: C
168. ANS: B
169. ANS: D
170. ANS: A
171. ANS: C
172. ANS: B
173. ANS: D
174. ANS: A
175. ANS: C

This Page Was Intentionally Left Blank

A Practical Study Guide For The Surgical Technologist Certification Exam

ALL QUESTIONS IN THIS MOCK EXAM REPRESENT A BREAK DOWN IN THE NUMBER OF QUESTIONS TO A SPECIFIC TOPIC AS INDICATED BY NBSTSA

MOCK CERTIFICATION EXAMINATION
PRACTICE EXAMINATION

DO NOT OPEN THE BOOK UNTIL READY TO BEGIN EXAM
CANDIDATE HAS 4 HOURS TO COMPLETE THIS EXAM
DO NOT WRITE IN THIS TEST BOOKLET

TEST BOOK 0002

BSTA Mock Exam Test 2

1. The needs or activities related to one's identification or interaction with another individual or group forms which component of the human being?
   a. social
   b. psychological
   c. physical
   d. physiological

2. If adult response is the norm, pediatric patients must be observed for which response?
   a. no variants in response
   b. paradoxical responses to some drugs
   c. increased crying
   d. decreased consciousness

3. Which term describes the following coping mechanism: "A patient tries to give excuses as to why he or she has a particular illness"?
   a. regression
   b. rationalization
   c. denial
   d. repression

4. The critical parameters for monitoring pediatric patients include all of the following EXCEPT _____.
   a. temperature
   b. urine output
   c. oxygenation
   d. turgor

5. Bleeding in a pediatric trauma patient must be controlled to prevent _____.
   a. brachial plexus injury
   b. infiltration
   c. distension
   d. severe hypovolemia

6. During abdominal procedures on patients who are obese, what procedure might additionally be performed due to newly identified pathology?
   a. pancreatectomy
   b. Whipple
   c. cholecystectomy
   d. splenectomy

7. Which disease is NOT an autoimmune disease?
   a. multiple sclerosis
   b. AIDS
   c. lupus erythematosus
   d. rheumatoid arthritis

8. When placing the pregnant surgical patient in the supine position, the circulating surgical technologist should place a small rolled pad or sheet under the right hip. This will help _____.
   a. take weight off of the vena cava
   b. make the patient more comfortable
   c. shift the uterus to gain better access to the abdominal contents
   d. prevent preterm labor

9. Emergency procedures on geriatric patients are associated with _____.
   a. better preoperative planning
   b. higher mortality
   c. trauma
   d. failure to minimize postoperative stress of hypothermia and hypoxemia

10. The _____ is the number one organ injured in a motor vehicle accident.
    a. heart
    b. liver
    c. spleen
    d. abdominal aorta

11. Why should cabinets and doors within the operating room be recessed into the wall?
    a. prevent injuries
    b. easy opening
    c. prevent dust accumulation
    d. cleaning purposes

12. When an electrical charge is in motion, it is referred to as a(n) _____.
    a. electrical current
    b. active current
    c. open current
    d. closed current

13. What is used to create a pathway for electrical current to be returned from the patient back to the ESU?
    a. Bovie cord
    b. grounding pad
    c. ground wire
    d. conducting gel

14. Which machine found in the decontamination room uses cavitation?
    a. ultrasonic washer
    b. washer sterilizer
    c. dry heat
    d. flash sterilizer

15. A unidirectional positive-pressure flow of air that captures microbes to be filtered is known as ____.
    a. negative airflow
    b. pressurized air
    c. laminar airflow
    d. sterile airflow

16. ____ means microbes and infection are absent.
    a. Sterile
    b. Surgically clean
    c. Decontaminated
    d. Disinfected

17. Fluid bottles may be recapped and reused under what conditions?
    a. The fluid is to be warmed.
    b. The bottle is sterile.
    c. The pourer is wearing gloves.
    d. None: the bottle may not be recapped.

18. The ____ is used to remove small organic particles and soil from areas of instruments that are difficult to clean manually.
    a. ultrasonic washer
    b. CUSA
    c. wire brush
    d. gas sterilizer

19. Which classification is given to bacteria that can survive in an environment with or without oxygen?
    a. facultative anaerobes
    b. capnophiles
    c. microaerophiles
    d. obligate anaerobes

20. Which is the most commonly transmitted bacteria in the operating room?
    a. *Candida albicans*
    b. *Corynebacterium jeikeium*
    c. *Staphylococcus aureus*
    d. *Streptococcus pneumoniae*

21. Which microorganism is capable of causing an UTI?
    a. *Staphylococcus aureus*
    b. *Staphylococcus epidermidis*
    c. *Streptococcus pyogenes*
    d. *Streptococcus agalactiae*

22. Gas gangrene and cellulitis is caused by which microorganism?
    a. *Klebsiella pneumoniae*
    b. *Pasteurella multocida*
    c. *Clostridium perfringens*
    d. *E. coli*

23. The scope used for visualization of a fetus in utero is called a(n) ____.
    a. laryngoscope
    b. fetoscope
    c. hysteroscope
    d. colonoscope

24. Sponges used for procedures requiring smaller incisions are called ____.
    a. laparotomy
    b. neurosurgical
    c. Raytec
    d. tonsil

25. A Tru-Cut needle is used ____.
    a. to obtain a biopsy
    b. during cardiovascular procedures
    c. to introduce angioplasty-guiding catheters
    d. to irrigate open arteries

26. Small, clear, plastic drapes with openings that are surrounded by an adhesive backing are called ____ drapes.
    a. incise
    b. isolation
    c. reusable
    d. aperture

27. Postoperative instrument handling involves all of the following steps EXCEPT ____.
    a. cleaning and decontamination
    b. reassembly
    c. preparation
    d. distribution

28. Curved needle holders are generally used during ____ procedures.
    a. orthopedic
    b. cardiovascular procedures
    c. gynecological
    d. plastic and reconstructive

29. While the STSR is passing instruments, the surgeon is focused on the ____.
    a. exchange
    b. procedure
    c. operating room setup
    d. anesthesia delivery

30. Items are counted in which order for every procedure?
    a. sharps, sponges, instruments
    b. instruments, sharps, sponges
    c. sponges, instruments, sharps
    d. sponges, sharps, instruments

31. Which term means loss of heat from the patient's body to the environment?
    a. convection
    b. radiation
    c. conduction
    d. evaporation

32. Which diagnostic imaging procedure allows the surgeon to view anatomic structures during the surgical procedure?
    a. conventional X-ray
    b. ultrasound
    c. fluoroscopy
    d. MRI

33. The display and recording of the electrical activity of skeletal muscle is called a(n) _____.
    a. EEG
    b. ECG
    c. EMG
    d. PET scan

34. Arterial saturation of hemoglobin with oxygen is measured with the use of _____.
    a. pulse oximetry
    b. capnography
    c. spirometry
    d. plethysmography

35. Correct placement of indwelling catheters, tubes, and drains may be verified by _____.
    a. radiography
    b. pulse oximetry
    c. auscultation
    d. endoscopy

36. Which diagnostic procedure uses high-frequency sound waves?
    a. MRI
    b. PET
    c. ultrasound
    d. CT

37. The beta cells of the islets of Langerhans are responsible for the production of _____.
    a. vitamin K
    b. glucagon
    c. insulin
    d. somatostatin

38. Nissen fundoplication is the procedure performed to correct a(n) _____.
    a. gastric ulcer
    b. inguinal hernia
    c. hiatal hernia
    d. ruptured tubal pregnancy

39. An end ileostomy is created from the ____.
    a. transverse colon
    b. descending colon
    c. terminal ileum
    d. sigmoid colon

40. Modified radical mastectomy involves removal of ____.
    a. the breast, axillary lymph nodes, and pectoral muscles
    b. the breast and axillary lymph nodes
    c. a wedge of breast tissue
    d. the breast

41. Which of the following describes the anatomic area that will be prepped for a laparotomy?
    a. midchest to midthighs and bilaterally
    b. chin to knees and bilaterally
    c. shoulders to hips and bilaterally
    d. midchest to iliac crests and bilaterally

42. Mastectomy is the removal of the ____.
    a. entire mammary breast
    b. entire breast and pectoral muscles
    c. entire breast, pectoral muscles, and axillary lymph nodes
    d. tumor only, preserving subcutaneous tissue for reconstruction

43. Roux-en-Y technique is most commonly used to repair a(n) ____.
    a. total gastrectomy
    b. colon resection
    c. cholecystectomy
    d. end-loop ileostomy

44. The pH of vaginal fluid is ____.
    a. acidic
    b. alkaline
    c. neutral
    d. base

45. The term *D and C* represents ____.
    a. disinfection and culture
    b. dilation and culture
    c. dilation and curettage
    d. desensitization and curettage

46. Cystocele is prolapse of the ____.
    a. bladder into the vaginal vault
    b. rectum into the vaginal vault
    c. uterus through the vagina
    d. intestine into the vaginal vault

47. A curette is a surgical instrument used to ____.
    a. dilate an opening
    b. marsupialize a cyst
    c. remove tissue by scraping
    d. provide traction

48. Which female gland secretes a lubricating mucoid substance?
    a. Cowper's gland
    b. pineal gland
    c. Bartholin's gland
    d. sudoriferous gland

49. What is the function of the iris?
    a. to alter the shape of the crystalline lens during accommodation
    b. to regulate the amount of light entering the eye through the pupil
    c. to produce tears
    d. to allow the optic nerve to carry visual impulses to the brain

50. Where are the lacrimal glands located?
    a. on the surface of the conjunctiva
    b. within the upper eyelids
    c. within the lower eyelids
    d. in the lateral corners of the eye

51. Why is Gelfoam used in ENT surgical procedures?
    a. achieve hemostasis
    b. reduce edema
    c. reduce high blood pressure
    d. increase body temperature

52. What does the term *apnea* mean?
    a. not breathing
    b. cardiac arrest
    c. deaf
    d. deviated septum

53. Panendoscopy may involve viewing of the ____.
    a. lungs
    b. stomach
    c. esophagus
    d. bronchi

54. What structures are removed during UPPP?
    a. tonsils, adenoids, uvula, portion of the soft palate
    b. adenoids, tongue, lingual tonsils, portion of the soft palate
    c. tonsils, adenoids, nasal cartilage, all of the soft palate
    d. adenoids, tonsils, tonsillar fossa, nasal cartilage

55. What is a major concern when operating on the parotid gland?
    a. inability to produce saliva post-op   c. carotid artery
    b. damage to the ossicles   d. facial nerve

56. During a tonsillectomy, which instrument can be used to put tension on the tonsil during dissection?
    a. Jensen Middleton   c. Rosen knife
    b. long Allis   d. Aufricht retractor

57. Crescent-shaped cartilage found in the TMJ and knee joints is the ____.
    a. sagittal   c. ramus
    b. symphysis   d. meniscus

58. Which of the following is an action of epinephrine?
    a. bronchodilation   c. analgesia
    b. vasoconstriction   d. anticoagulant

59. Which radiographic view shows the hard palate, nasal septum, orbital floor, and zygoma?
    a. Waters' view   c. panoramic view
    b. Caldwell view   d. lateral facial view

60. All are true regarding throat packs EXCEPT that ____.
    a. throat packs consist of rolled gauze that contains a radiopaque marker.
    b. throat packs are kept dry and used to prevent oral secretions, irrigation fluid, blood, and bone or tooth fragments from becoming lodged in the pharynx
    c. the throat pack should be removed prior to extubation
    d. the throat pack should be included in the formal count

61. Which muscle is responsible for flexing the hand at the wrist?
    a. abductor pollicis brevis   c. palmaris longus
    b. extensor digitorum   d. adductor pollicis

62. A cosmetic procedure performed on the eyelid is a(n) ____.
    a. blepharoplasty   c. rhinoplasty
    b. suction lipectomy   d. augmentation

127. The two bones that make up the posterior nasal septum are the:
    a. nasal and lacrimal
    b. inferior nasal choncae and vomer
    c. vomer and ethmoid
    d. ethmoid and sphenoid

128. Which of the following is the most serious or life-threatening:
    a. deviated nasal septum
    b. sinusitis
    c. damaged cribriform plate
    d. damaged or cleft palate
    e. ruptured bursae

129. "Articulations" refers to:
    a. broken bones
    b. the study of individual bones
    c. bone growth and remodeling
    d. structures on bones where muscles attach
    e. joints

130. Which of the following bone is not part of the cranium:
    a. sphenoid
    b. palatine
    c. ethmoid
    d. occipital

131. Which of the following is not part of the axial skeleton:
    a. femur
    b. sternum
    c. mandible
    d. sacrum

132. The "Hunchback" of Notre Dame probably suffered from:
    a. cleft palate
    b. scoliosis
    c. kyphosis
    d. lordosis
    e. spina bifida

121. These structures are at the center of compact bone lamellae and carry blood vessels along the bone length:
    a. Haversian canals
    b. canaliculi
    c. perforating canals
    d. osteocytes
    e. lacunae

122. The cell type that is responsible for maintaining bone matrix once it has formed is:
    a. osteoclasts
    b. chondrocytes
    c. osteocytes
    d. fibroblasts
    e. osteoblasts

123. Soft connective tissue membranes between the cranial bones at birth are:
    a. an indication of microcephaly
    b. frontal sinuses
    c. epiphyseal plates
    d. cribriform plates
    e. fontanelles

124. Endochondral and intramembranous are two mechanisms of:
    a. bone remodeling
    b. embryonic skeletal ossification
    c. controlling blood calcium levels
    d. cartilage synthesis

125. Which of the following is not a cranial suture:
    a. epiphyseal
    b. lambdoidal
    c. coronal
    d. sagittal
    e. squamous

126. The two pairs of bones that make up the hard palate are the right and left:
    a. zygomatic and temporal
    b. palatine and maxillae
    c. maxillae and zygomatic
    d. maxillae and mandible

116. Which of the following bones is considered a sesamoid bone:
    a. sternum
    b. ethmoid
    c. femur
    d. patella
    e. phalanx

117. These two components in bone are responsible for the hardness and pliability of bone:
    a. osteoclasts & collagen
    b. mineralized salts & osteocytes
    c. mineralized salts & collagen
    d. collagen & elastic fibers
    e. collagen & mesenchyme

118. A fracture in the shaft of a long bone would be a break in the:
    a. epiphysis
    b. metaphysis
    c. diaphysis
    d. epiphyseal plate
    e. mesenchyme

119. Yellow marrow consists of:
    a. osteoprogenitor cells
    b. blood cell progenitor cells
    c. hyaline cartilage
    d. adipose
    e. spongy bone

120. Chondroblasts produce:
    a. basement membranes
    b. bone matrix
    c. cartilage matrix
    d. mesothelium
    e. endothelium

108. Negligence is a breach of duty and is defined as ____.
    a. an omission
    b. perjury
    c. tort
    d. larceny

109. When taking hot surgical instruments from a steam autoclave, the surgical technologist is responsible for cooling the instruments with ____.
    a. alcohol
    b. sterile saline
    c. glutaraldehyde
    d. sterile water

110. What must be done to electrical devices in the operating room to prevent the risk of burns to the patient?
    a. grounded properly
    b. turned off prior to use
    c. tested frequently
    d. both A and C

111. Loss or mishandling of a specimen could be considered negligence and could result in ____.
    a. another surgical procedure
    b. improper specimen preparation
    c. improper specimen analysis
    d. all of the above

112. The only method used to ensure the sterility of items is ____.
    a. chemical indicator strips
    b. biological indicators
    c. mechanical indicators
    d. Bowie-Dick test

113. Implied consent may apply when ____.
    a. consulting physicians agree
    b. the patient is conscious
    c. conditions are discovered during surgery
    d. the patient is an emancipated minor

114. In the health care field, the term ____ is used broadly to refer to the placing of information into a patient's medical record.
    a. register
    b. remodeling
    c. documenting
    d. diagram

115. The dense connective tissue covering outer surface of bone diaphyses is termed:
    a. perichondrium
    b. periosteum
    c. endosteum
    d. exofibrium
    e. articular cartilage

100. The room where patients are "recovered" immediately following surgery is known as the _____.
    a. JCAHO
    b. CPSD
    c. PACU
    d. NCIU

101. Which of the following is a reason a patient may be extubated in the recovery room instead of the operating room suite?
    a. tachypnea
    b. tachycardia
    c. Patient can breathe unassisted.
    d. Patient cannot breathe unassisted.

102. When stainless steel instruments are manually cleaned, a(n) _____ should be used to avoid scratching the surface of the instrument.
    a. circular motion
    b. abrasive cleanser
    c. wire brush
    d. back-and-forth motion

103. What is a limitation of using water as a presoaking solution?
    a. ineffective at removing dried debris
    b. too expensive
    c. not readily available
    d. not a sterile solution

104. Why should saline NOT be used to clean stainless steel surgical instruments?
    a. Saline is not virucidal.
    b. Salt will pit the stainless steel.
    c. Saline is not sterile.
    d. Saline is expensive.

105. An enzyme is usually used as a(n) _____.
    a. sterilant
    b. disinfectant
    c. antiseptic
    d. soaking solution

106. Which of the following reflects the basic values for health care practice?
    a. laws
    b. standards
    c. guidelines
    d. all of the above

107. Accountability is defined as a(n) _____.
    a. disclosure
    b. obligation
    c. threat
    d. evaluation

93. The sphenoid bone forms ____.
    a. a small portion of the sides and floor of the cranium
    b. a large portion of the sides and roof of the cranium
    c. portions of the base of the cranium, sides of the skull, and base and sides for the orbits
    d. portions of the roof and walls of the nasal cavity, the floor of the cranium, and walls of the orbits

94. The midbrain is located just below the ____.
    a. hypothalamus
    b. pituitary
    c. thalamus
    d. pons

95. What nerve controls the voluntary muscles of the pharynx, larynx, palate, sternocleidomastoid, and trapezius?
    a. accessory
    b. hypoglossal
    c. glossopharyngeal
    d. abducens

96. What name is given to the room in the surgery department that contains sinks for gross decontamination of instruments?
    a. substerile
    b. sterile storage
    c. decontamination
    d. instrument

97. The term *PACU* refers to the ____.
    a. post ambulatory care unit
    b. primary anesthesia care unit
    c. post anesthesia care unit
    d. preoperative ambulatory care unit

98. Permanent surgical specimens are usually sent to the pathologist in ____.
    a. saline
    b. formalin
    c. a dry container
    d. a moist towel

99. Operating room walls should have which characteristic?
    a. surgically clean and tiled
    b. bright white to create a sense of sterility
    c. easy to clean with an antimicrobial solution
    d. mini blinds for patient privacy

85. Which type of needle is appropriate for closing a blood vessel?
    a. blunt
    b. conventional cutting
    c. taper
    d. side cutting

86. The external iliac arteries branch into the ____ arteries.
    a. internal iliac
    b. femoral
    c. celiac
    d. brachial

87. Which drug is used to suppress arterial vasospasm?
    a. Avitene
    b. Hypaque
    c. papaverine
    d. heparin

88. The ____ serves as a relay station for sensory impulses by channeling them to appropriate regions of the cortex for interpretation.
    a. hypothalamus
    b. thalamus
    c. basal ganglia
    d. pons

89. The medulla oblongata controls which visceral activity?
    a. cardiac
    b. vasomotor
    c. respiratory
    d. all of the above

90. A ventricular shunt can be placed distally in the ____.
    a. ventricle or the perineum
    b. atrium or the peritoneal cavity
    c. atrium or the thoracic cavity
    d. ventricle or the aorta

91. What is the best temperature for irrigation used on the brain?
    a. cold
    b. hot
    c. room temperature
    d. body temperature

92. Which statement is NOT correct regarding the placement of the bone flap?
    a. The bone flap is placed after the muscle layer is closed with an absorbable suture.
    b. The bone flap is placed after the dura has been securely closed.
    c. The bone flap remains on the sterile field throughout the procedure, typically in a solution of antibiotic saline.
    d. The bone flap can be fixated to the skull with the use of titanium miniplates and screws.

78. Which mechanical device is designed for circulatory support after cardiac procedures?
    a. cell saver
    b. Fogarty embolectomy catheter
    c. intra-aortic balloon pump
    d. arterial line

79. The trachea divides at the _____ into right and left bronchi.
    a. glottis
    b. carina
    c. epiglottis
    d. bronchioles

80. Symptomatic lesions of the mediastinum are malignant in _____% of all patients?
    a. 50
    b. 20
    c. 60
    d. 10

81. For the posterolateral position, the operating room personnel should have which of the following available?
    a. 2-inch adhesive tape
    b. beanbag
    c. extra arm boards
    d. shoulder rests

82. Which veins receive blood from the brain, meninges, and deeper regions of the face and neck?
    a. brachiocephalic
    b. external jugular
    c. internal jugular
    d. common carotid

83. For an aortofemoral bypass, which statement is NOT correct?
    a. The patient will be prepped from midchest to midthigh and as far as possible on each side.
    b. The circulator should ensure that blood is available for the patient.
    c. The arterial incision is made with a #10 blade on a long #3 handle.
    d. 2-0 or 3-0 silk ties can be used to ligate larger, deeper vessels.

84. What graft material is not recommended to be used in the popliteal space?
    a. PTFE
    b. porous Dacron graft
    c. saphenous vein
    d. specialized knitted velour Dacron graft

70. The right kidney is located slightly lower than the left, due to the ____.
    a. liver
    b. pancreas
    c. spleen
    d. stomach

71. The kidneys are bounded by the ____ muscles on the medial side.
    a. detrusor
    b. cremaster
    c. psoas
    d. transverse abdominal

72. If the ureters are difficult to identify when the bladder is opened, intravenous ____ may facilitate locating the orifices.
    a. methylene blue
    b. gentian violet
    c. indigo carmine
    d. omnipaque

73. A softening of adult bone due to a disorder in calcium and phosphorus metabolism is called ____.
    a. osteochondritis
    b. osteogenesis
    c. osteomalacia
    d. osteonecrosis

74. Which of the following constitutes the anterior portion of the coxal bone?
    a. ischium
    b. ilium
    c. sacrum
    d. pubis

75. Which style of cast is applied to the trunk, around the affected leg, and around half of the unaffected leg?
    a. long-leg cast
    b. cylinder cast
    c. hip spica
    d. body jacket

76. The coronary arteries arise from the ____.
    a. aorta
    b. vena cavae
    c. pulmonary artery
    d. subclavian artery

77. What medical term refers to the abnormal accumulation of air in the pleural cavity?
    a. pneumocentesis
    b. pneumothorax
    c. pleural effusion
    d. thoracic outlet syndrome

63. Which of the following best describes the area of the skin preparation for a reduction mammoplasty?
    a. chest and breast, shoulders to xiphoid process
    b. chest and breast, chin to xiphoid process including axilla
    c. chest and breast, chin to hips including axilla
    d. chest and breast, shoulders to hips

64. How many phalanges are in a normal hand?
    a. 12
    b. 14
    c. 16
    d. 18

65. Which of the following is a topical anesthetic inserted into the nose prior to a plastic nasal procedure?
    a. bupivacaine
    b. Tetracaine
    c. meperidine
    d. fentanyl

66. Which type of flap allows the tissue to be transferred to remain attached to its blood supply?
    a. free flap
    b. pedicle flap
    c. skin tag
    d. de Quervain's

67. Which type of instrument will be attached to the Mayo stand during a cleft palate repair?
    a. Cottle elevator
    b. Bookwalter
    c. Weitlaner
    d. self-retaining mouth gag

68. Which portion of the renal tubule system is responsible for increasing the surface area for enhanced absorption and secretion?
    a. Bowman's capsule
    b. distal convoluted tubule
    c. loop of Henle
    d. proximal convoluted tubule

69. What surgical instrument is used to remove tissue fragments from within the bladder during a transurethral resection of the prostate (TURP)?
    a. resectoscope
    b. urethrotome
    c. Ellik evacuator
    d. urethral forceps

133. Incomplete closure of the vertebral column results in:
    a. spina bifida
    b. scoliosis
    c. sinusitis
    d. kyphosis
    e. lordosis

134. The thickened cartilage "cushions" found in the knee and vertebral joints that absorb compression are:
    a. the menisci
    b. the bursae
    c. the ligaments
    d. the synovial capsules
    e. epiphyseal plates

135. Which of the following does **not** describe synovial joints:
    a. bones held together by cartilage
    b. joint surfaces of bones covered with articulating cartilage
    c. has joint cavity
    d. has 2-layered joint capsule
    e. most freely movable of joints

136. A ligament running along the side of the knee joint is a:
    a. cruciate
    b. bursae
    c. collateral
    d. patellar

137. Which of the following is least likely to require arthroscopic surgery:
    a. removal of a torn meniscus in the knee
    b. removal of torn articular cartilage in the knee
    c. repair of a torn lateral collateral ligament in the knee
    d. repair of a torn anterior cruciate ligament in the knee

138. The Haversian (central) canal in each osteon contains:
    a. chondroitin sulfate
    b. hydroxyapatite
    c. osteoblasts
    d. blood vessels
    e. synovial fluid

139. This hormone stimulates the breakdown of bone and the increase in blood calcium levels:
    a. growth hormone
    b. estrogen
    c. parathyroid hormone
    d. calcitonin

140. The space in the middle of the thoracic cavity where the heart resides is the:
    a. pericardial cavity
    b. pericardium
    c. pleural cavity
    d. mediastinum
    e. dorsal cavity

141. Blood returning from the lungs enters the heart through the:
    a. pulmonary semilunar valve
    b. mitral valve
    c. right ventricle
    d. left atrium
    e. vena cava

142. During ventricular systole:
    a. the atria are contracting
    b. the AV valves are closed
    c. the pressure inside the ventricles is less than in the atria
    d. the mitral valve is closed
    e. blood is ejected into the atria

143. A vertical plane through the body dividing it into right and left is termed:
    a. sagittal
    b. lateral
    c. transverse
    d. frontal

144. The anatomical position is characterized by all of the following except:
    a. palms facing posterior
    b. thumbs pointing laterally
    c. face pointing anteriorly
    d. body standing upright

145. The number of microbes or organic debris that exist at a given time is referred to as ____.
    a. contamination
    b. asepsis
    c. bioburden
    d. sterilization

146. Which term is used to describe "the multiplication of organisms in tissue"?
    a. nosocomial
    b. infection
    c. cross contamination
    d. culture

147. *Escherichia coli* normally resides in the lumen of the ____.
    a. esophagus
    b. trachea
    c. intestine
    d. urethra

148. Bacilli are typically found to be in the shape of ____.
    a. spirals
    b. rounds
    c. L forms
    d. rods

149. Bacteria that require oxygen to sustain life are called ____.
    a. anaerobic
    b. aerobic
    c. rods
    d. protozoa

150. Which pathogen leads in the percentage of surgical site infections?
    a. *Staphylococcus aureus*
    b. *Cryptosporidium*
    c. *Candida albicans*
    d. *Pseudomonas aeruginosa*

151. What dormant structure can some bacteria form to survive adverse environmental conditions?
    a. vegetative state
    b. spore
    c. spirillum
    d. lysogenic

152. A nonliving particle that is completely reliant on the host cell for survival is called a ____.
    a. bacteria
    b. fungus
    c. protozoa
    d. virus

153. A bloodborne pathogen that puts health care workers at particular risk is _____.
    a. hepatitis C
    b. *Staphylococcus aureus*
    c. *Mycobacterium tuberculosis*
    d. all helminths

154. Microbes that live on the skin and inside the human body are referred to as _____.
    a. symbiotic
    b. indigenous
    c. anaerobic
    d. aerobic

155. Drug administered within a joint is _____.
    a. subcutaneous
    b. intravenous
    c. intra-articular
    d. dermal

156. Drugs with a high potential to cause psychological or physical dependence and abuse are called _____.
    a. over-the-counter medications
    b. chemical substances
    c. prescription medications
    d. controlled substances

157. The main function of the liver in metabolism is to _____.
    a. break down drug molecules
    b. transport the drug
    c. absorb the drug
    d. distribute the drug

158. Pharmacodynamics describes the interaction of the _____.
    a. target organ and circulatory system
    b. drugs and capillaries
    c. heart and lungs
    d. drug molecules and target cells

159. The time it takes from the administration of a drug until its action becomes evident refers to _____.
    a. transition period
    b. onset
    c. duration
    d. function

160. What theory states that the active substance in a drug has an affinity for a specific chemical constituent of a cell?
    a. drug-enzyme interaction
    b. drug-receptor interaction
    c. membrane interaction
    d. antagonistic drug interaction

161. Which of the following focuses on altering the patient's level of consciousness and minimizing pain and awareness?
    a. conduction blockade
    b. general anesthesia
    c. hypnosis
    d. amnesia

162. Which of the following is the generic name for Marcaine?
    a. Pitocin
    b. xylocaine
    c. bupivacaine
    d. Novocain

163. Which agents selectively interrupt the associative pathways of the brain?
    a. opioids
    b. dissociative
    c. induction
    d. Tranquilizers

164. When stainless steel instruments are manually cleaned, a(n) ____ should be used to avoid scratching the surface of the instrument.
    a. circular motion
    b. abrasive cleanser
    c. wire brush
    d. back-and-forth motion

165. What is a limitation of using water as a presoaking solution?
    a. ineffective at removing dried debris
    b. too expensive
    c. not readily available
    d. not a sterile solution

166. The ultrasonic washer is an example of a ____.
    a. sterilizer
    b. mechanical decontamination unit
    c. physical decontamination method
    d. bioburden

167. The washer decontaminator does NOT render the instruments ____.
    a. sterile
    b. surgically clean
    c. disinfected
    d. safe to handle

168. At the end of the washer sterilization cycle, instruments are NOT considered ____.
    a. safe to handle
    b. appropriate for use on the patient
    c. ready for assembly into sets
    d. ready for processing

169. An intermediate level of disinfection may be appropriate for ____.
    a. semicritical items
    b. critical items
    c. microsurgical instruments
    d. GI instruments

170. Physical factors that affect the efficiency of disinfection are ____.
    a. time, temperature, pressure
    b. humidity, temperature, pressure
    c. temperature, gross debris, bioburden
    d. temperature, bioburden, time

171. To prevent the formation of condensate in nested basins (double basin), what must be done?
    a. Separate the basins with a towel.
    b. Do not nest the basins.
    c. Ensure metal-to-metal contact.
    d. Separate the basins with a plastic sheet.

172. Which would be best suited for reprocessing surgical instruments exposed to clostridium?
    a. glutaraldehyde
    b. cidex
    c. isopropyl alcohol
    d. pre-vac

173. The process used to relieve pain during surgical intervention refers to ____ administration.
    a. tranquilizer
    b. anesthesia
    c. narcotics
    d. neuromuscular block

174. Which risk is not associated with general anesthesia?
    a. cardiac arrest
    b. shock
    c. muscle relaxation
    d. allergic reaction

175. Demerol, Sublimaze, Sufenta, and Alfenta are examples of ____.
    a. opioids
    b. dissociative agents
    c. narcotic antagonists
    d. hypnotic agents

THIS PAGE IS LEFT INTENTIONALY BLANK

A Practical Study Guide For The Surgical Technologist Certification Exam

NBSTA Mock Exam
NAME: _____ DATE: _____ EXAM NUMBER____

MULTIPLE CHOICE

#		#		#		#	
1.	Ⓐ Ⓑ Ⓒ Ⓓ Ⓔ	49.	Ⓐ Ⓑ Ⓒ Ⓓ Ⓔ	97.	Ⓐ Ⓑ Ⓒ Ⓓ Ⓔ	145.	Ⓐ Ⓑ Ⓒ Ⓓ Ⓔ
2.	Ⓐ Ⓑ Ⓒ Ⓓ Ⓔ	50.	Ⓐ Ⓑ Ⓒ Ⓓ Ⓔ	98.	Ⓐ Ⓑ Ⓒ Ⓓ Ⓔ	146.	Ⓐ Ⓑ Ⓒ Ⓓ Ⓔ
3.	Ⓐ Ⓑ Ⓒ Ⓓ Ⓔ	51.	Ⓐ Ⓑ Ⓒ Ⓓ Ⓔ	99.	Ⓐ Ⓑ Ⓒ Ⓓ Ⓔ	147.	Ⓐ Ⓑ Ⓒ Ⓓ Ⓔ
4.	Ⓐ Ⓑ Ⓒ Ⓓ Ⓔ	52.	Ⓐ Ⓑ Ⓒ Ⓓ Ⓔ	100.	Ⓐ Ⓑ Ⓒ Ⓓ Ⓔ	148.	Ⓐ Ⓑ Ⓒ Ⓓ Ⓔ
5.	Ⓐ Ⓑ Ⓒ Ⓓ Ⓔ	53.	Ⓐ Ⓑ Ⓒ Ⓓ Ⓔ	101.	Ⓐ Ⓑ Ⓒ Ⓓ Ⓔ	149.	Ⓐ Ⓑ Ⓒ Ⓓ Ⓔ
6.	Ⓐ Ⓑ Ⓒ Ⓓ Ⓔ	54.	Ⓐ Ⓑ Ⓒ Ⓓ Ⓔ	102.	Ⓐ Ⓑ Ⓒ Ⓓ Ⓔ	150.	Ⓐ Ⓑ Ⓒ Ⓓ Ⓔ
7.	Ⓐ Ⓑ Ⓒ Ⓓ Ⓔ	55.	Ⓐ Ⓑ Ⓒ Ⓓ Ⓔ	103.	Ⓐ Ⓑ Ⓒ Ⓓ Ⓔ	151.	Ⓐ Ⓑ Ⓒ Ⓓ Ⓔ
8.	Ⓐ Ⓑ Ⓒ Ⓓ Ⓔ	56.	Ⓐ Ⓑ Ⓒ Ⓓ Ⓔ	104.	Ⓐ Ⓑ Ⓒ Ⓓ Ⓔ	152.	Ⓐ Ⓑ Ⓒ Ⓓ Ⓔ
9.	Ⓐ Ⓑ Ⓒ Ⓓ Ⓔ	57.	Ⓐ Ⓑ Ⓒ Ⓓ Ⓔ	105.	Ⓐ Ⓑ Ⓒ Ⓓ Ⓔ	153.	Ⓐ Ⓑ Ⓒ Ⓓ Ⓔ
10.	Ⓐ Ⓑ Ⓒ Ⓓ Ⓔ	58.	Ⓐ Ⓑ Ⓒ Ⓓ Ⓔ	106.	Ⓐ Ⓑ Ⓒ Ⓓ Ⓔ	154.	Ⓐ Ⓑ Ⓒ Ⓓ Ⓔ
11.	Ⓐ Ⓑ Ⓒ Ⓓ Ⓔ	59.	Ⓐ Ⓑ Ⓒ Ⓓ Ⓔ	107.	Ⓐ Ⓑ Ⓒ Ⓓ Ⓔ	155.	Ⓐ Ⓑ Ⓒ Ⓓ Ⓔ
12.	Ⓐ Ⓑ Ⓒ Ⓓ Ⓔ	60.	Ⓐ Ⓑ Ⓒ Ⓓ Ⓔ	108.	Ⓐ Ⓑ Ⓒ Ⓓ Ⓔ	156.	Ⓐ Ⓑ Ⓒ Ⓓ Ⓔ
13.	Ⓐ Ⓑ Ⓒ Ⓓ Ⓔ	61.	Ⓐ Ⓑ Ⓒ Ⓓ Ⓔ	109.	Ⓐ Ⓑ Ⓒ Ⓓ Ⓔ	157.	Ⓐ Ⓑ Ⓒ Ⓓ Ⓔ
14.	Ⓐ Ⓑ Ⓒ Ⓓ Ⓔ	62.	Ⓐ Ⓑ Ⓒ Ⓓ Ⓔ	110.	Ⓐ Ⓑ Ⓒ Ⓓ Ⓔ	158.	Ⓐ Ⓑ Ⓒ Ⓓ Ⓔ
15.	Ⓐ Ⓑ Ⓒ Ⓓ Ⓔ	63.	Ⓐ Ⓑ Ⓒ Ⓓ Ⓔ	111.	Ⓐ Ⓑ Ⓒ Ⓓ Ⓔ	159.	Ⓐ Ⓑ Ⓒ Ⓓ Ⓔ
16.	Ⓐ Ⓑ Ⓒ Ⓓ Ⓔ	64.	Ⓐ Ⓑ Ⓒ Ⓓ Ⓔ	112.	Ⓐ Ⓑ Ⓒ Ⓓ Ⓔ	160.	Ⓐ Ⓑ Ⓒ Ⓓ Ⓔ
17.	Ⓐ Ⓑ Ⓒ Ⓓ Ⓔ	65.	Ⓐ Ⓑ Ⓒ Ⓓ Ⓔ	113.	Ⓐ Ⓑ Ⓒ Ⓓ Ⓔ	161.	Ⓐ Ⓑ Ⓒ Ⓓ Ⓔ
18.	Ⓐ Ⓑ Ⓒ Ⓓ Ⓔ	66.	Ⓐ Ⓑ Ⓒ Ⓓ Ⓔ	114.	Ⓐ Ⓑ Ⓒ Ⓓ Ⓔ	162.	Ⓐ Ⓑ Ⓒ Ⓓ Ⓔ
19.	Ⓐ Ⓑ Ⓒ Ⓓ Ⓔ	67.	Ⓐ Ⓑ Ⓒ Ⓓ Ⓔ	115.	Ⓐ Ⓑ Ⓒ Ⓓ Ⓔ	163.	Ⓐ Ⓑ Ⓒ Ⓓ Ⓔ
20.	Ⓐ Ⓑ Ⓒ Ⓓ Ⓔ	68.	Ⓐ Ⓑ Ⓒ Ⓓ Ⓔ	116.	Ⓐ Ⓑ Ⓒ Ⓓ Ⓔ	164.	Ⓐ Ⓑ Ⓒ Ⓓ Ⓔ
21.	Ⓐ Ⓑ Ⓒ Ⓓ Ⓔ	69.	Ⓐ Ⓑ Ⓒ Ⓓ Ⓔ	117.	Ⓐ Ⓑ Ⓒ Ⓓ Ⓔ	165.	Ⓐ Ⓑ Ⓒ Ⓓ Ⓔ
22.	Ⓐ Ⓑ Ⓒ Ⓓ Ⓔ	70.	Ⓐ Ⓑ Ⓒ Ⓓ Ⓔ	118.	Ⓐ Ⓑ Ⓒ Ⓓ Ⓔ	166.	Ⓐ Ⓑ Ⓒ Ⓓ Ⓔ
23.	Ⓐ Ⓑ Ⓒ Ⓓ Ⓔ	71.	Ⓐ Ⓑ Ⓒ Ⓓ Ⓔ	119.	Ⓐ Ⓑ Ⓒ Ⓓ Ⓔ	167.	Ⓐ Ⓑ Ⓒ Ⓓ Ⓔ
24.	Ⓐ Ⓑ Ⓒ Ⓓ Ⓔ	72.	Ⓐ Ⓑ Ⓒ Ⓓ Ⓔ	120.	Ⓐ Ⓑ Ⓒ Ⓓ Ⓔ	168.	Ⓐ Ⓑ Ⓒ Ⓓ Ⓔ
25.	Ⓐ Ⓑ Ⓒ Ⓓ Ⓔ	73.	Ⓐ Ⓑ Ⓒ Ⓓ Ⓔ	121.	Ⓐ Ⓑ Ⓒ Ⓓ Ⓔ	169.	Ⓐ Ⓑ Ⓒ Ⓓ Ⓔ
26.	Ⓐ Ⓑ Ⓒ Ⓓ Ⓔ	74.	Ⓐ Ⓑ Ⓒ Ⓓ Ⓔ	122.	Ⓐ Ⓑ Ⓒ Ⓓ Ⓔ	170.	Ⓐ Ⓑ Ⓒ Ⓓ Ⓔ
27.	Ⓐ Ⓑ Ⓒ Ⓓ Ⓔ	75.	Ⓐ Ⓑ Ⓒ Ⓓ Ⓔ	123.	Ⓐ Ⓑ Ⓒ Ⓓ Ⓔ	171.	Ⓐ Ⓑ Ⓒ Ⓓ Ⓔ
28.	Ⓐ Ⓑ Ⓒ Ⓓ Ⓔ	76.	Ⓐ Ⓑ Ⓒ Ⓓ Ⓔ	124.	Ⓐ Ⓑ Ⓒ Ⓓ Ⓔ	172.	Ⓐ Ⓑ Ⓒ Ⓓ Ⓔ
29.	Ⓐ Ⓑ Ⓒ Ⓓ Ⓔ	77.	Ⓐ Ⓑ Ⓒ Ⓓ Ⓔ	125.	Ⓐ Ⓑ Ⓒ Ⓓ Ⓔ	173.	Ⓐ Ⓑ Ⓒ Ⓓ Ⓔ
30.	Ⓐ Ⓑ Ⓒ Ⓓ Ⓔ	78.	Ⓐ Ⓑ Ⓒ Ⓓ Ⓔ	126.	Ⓐ Ⓑ Ⓒ Ⓓ Ⓔ	174.	Ⓐ Ⓑ Ⓒ Ⓓ Ⓔ
31.	Ⓐ Ⓑ Ⓒ Ⓓ Ⓔ	79.	Ⓐ Ⓑ Ⓒ Ⓓ Ⓔ	127.	Ⓐ Ⓑ Ⓒ Ⓓ Ⓔ	175.	Ⓐ Ⓑ Ⓒ Ⓓ Ⓔ
32.	Ⓐ Ⓑ Ⓒ Ⓓ Ⓔ	80.	Ⓐ Ⓑ Ⓒ Ⓓ Ⓔ	128.	Ⓐ Ⓑ Ⓒ Ⓓ Ⓔ		
33.	Ⓐ Ⓑ Ⓒ Ⓓ Ⓔ	81.	Ⓐ Ⓑ Ⓒ Ⓓ Ⓔ	129.	Ⓐ Ⓑ Ⓒ Ⓓ Ⓔ		
34.	Ⓐ Ⓑ Ⓒ Ⓓ Ⓔ	82.	Ⓐ Ⓑ Ⓒ Ⓓ Ⓔ	130.	Ⓐ Ⓑ Ⓒ Ⓓ Ⓔ		
35.	Ⓐ Ⓑ Ⓒ Ⓓ Ⓔ	83.	Ⓐ Ⓑ Ⓒ Ⓓ Ⓔ	131.	Ⓐ Ⓑ Ⓒ Ⓓ Ⓔ		
36.	Ⓐ Ⓑ Ⓒ Ⓓ Ⓔ	84.	Ⓐ Ⓑ Ⓒ Ⓓ Ⓔ	132.	Ⓐ Ⓑ Ⓒ Ⓓ Ⓔ		
37.	Ⓐ Ⓑ Ⓒ Ⓓ Ⓔ	85.	Ⓐ Ⓑ Ⓒ Ⓓ Ⓔ	133.	Ⓐ Ⓑ Ⓒ Ⓓ Ⓔ		
38.	Ⓐ Ⓑ Ⓒ Ⓓ Ⓔ	86.	Ⓐ Ⓑ Ⓒ Ⓓ Ⓔ	134.	Ⓐ Ⓑ Ⓒ Ⓓ Ⓔ		
39.	Ⓐ Ⓑ Ⓒ Ⓓ Ⓔ	87.	Ⓐ Ⓑ Ⓒ Ⓓ Ⓔ	135.	Ⓐ Ⓑ Ⓒ Ⓓ Ⓔ		
40.	Ⓐ Ⓑ Ⓒ Ⓓ Ⓔ	88.	Ⓐ Ⓑ Ⓒ Ⓓ Ⓔ	136.	Ⓐ Ⓑ Ⓒ Ⓓ Ⓔ		
41.	Ⓐ Ⓑ Ⓒ Ⓓ Ⓔ	89.	Ⓐ Ⓑ Ⓒ Ⓓ Ⓔ	137.	Ⓐ Ⓑ Ⓒ Ⓓ Ⓔ		
42.	Ⓐ Ⓑ Ⓒ Ⓓ Ⓔ	90.	Ⓐ Ⓑ Ⓒ Ⓓ Ⓔ	138.	Ⓐ Ⓑ Ⓒ Ⓓ Ⓔ		
43.	Ⓐ Ⓑ Ⓒ Ⓓ Ⓔ	91.	Ⓐ Ⓑ Ⓒ Ⓓ Ⓔ	139.	Ⓐ Ⓑ Ⓒ Ⓓ Ⓔ		
44.	Ⓐ Ⓑ Ⓒ Ⓓ Ⓔ	92.	Ⓐ Ⓑ Ⓒ Ⓓ Ⓔ	140.	Ⓐ Ⓑ Ⓒ Ⓓ Ⓔ		
45.	Ⓐ Ⓑ Ⓒ Ⓓ Ⓔ	93.	Ⓐ Ⓑ Ⓒ Ⓓ Ⓔ	141.	Ⓐ Ⓑ Ⓒ Ⓓ Ⓔ		
46.	Ⓐ Ⓑ Ⓒ Ⓓ Ⓔ	94.	Ⓐ Ⓑ Ⓒ Ⓓ Ⓔ	142.	Ⓐ Ⓑ Ⓒ Ⓓ Ⓔ		
47.	Ⓐ Ⓑ Ⓒ Ⓓ Ⓔ	95.	Ⓐ Ⓑ Ⓒ Ⓓ Ⓔ	143.	Ⓐ Ⓑ Ⓒ Ⓓ Ⓔ		
48.	Ⓐ Ⓑ Ⓒ Ⓓ Ⓔ	96.	Ⓐ Ⓑ Ⓒ Ⓓ Ⓔ	144.	Ⓐ Ⓑ Ⓒ Ⓓ Ⓔ		

NBSTSA MOCK CERTIFICATION EXAM TEST 2

Answer Section

MULTIPLE CHOICE

1. ANS:A	*The Surgical Patient*

2. ANS:B	*The Surgical Patient*

3. ANS:B	*The Surgical Patient*

4. ANS:D	*Special Populations*

5. ANS:D	*Special Populations*

6. ANS:C	*Special Populations*

7. ANS:B	*Special Populations*

8. ANS:A	*Special Populations*

9. ANS:B	*Special Populations*

10. ANS:C	*Special Populations*

11. ANS:C	*Physical Environment and Safety Standards*

12. ANS:A	*Physical Environment and Safety Standards*

13. ANS:B	*Physical Environment and Safety Standards*

14. ANS:A	*Physical Environment and Safety Standards*

15. ANS:C	*Physical Environment and Safety Standards*

16. ANS:A	*Asepsis and Sterile Technique*

17. ANS:D   Asepsis and Sterile Technique

18. ANS:A   Asepsis and Sterile Technique

19. ANS:A   Asepsis and Sterile Technique

20. ANS:C   Asepsis and Sterile Technique

21. ANS:B   Asepsis and Sterile Technique

22. ANS:C   Asepsis and Sterile Technique

23. ANS:B   Instrumentation, Equipment, and Supplies

24. ANS:C   Instrumentation, Equipment, and Supplies

25. ANS:A   Instrumentation, Equipment, and Supplies

26. ANS:D   Instrumentation, Equipment, and Supplies

27. ANS:D   Instrumentation, Equipment, and Supplies

28. ANS:C   Instrumentation, Equipment, and Supplies

29. ANS:B   Surgical Case Management

30. ANS:D   Surgical Case Management

31. ANS:B   Surgical Case Management

32. ANS:C   Diagnostic Procedures

33. ANS:C   Diagnostic Procedures

34. ANS:A   Diagnostic Procedures

35. ANS:A   Diagnostic Procedures
36. ANS:C   Diagnostic Procedures
37. ANS:C   General Surgery
38. ANS:C   General Surgery
39. ANS:C   General Surgery
40. ANS:B   General Surgery
41. ANS:A   General Surgery
42. ANS:A   General Surgery
43. ANS:A   General Surgery
44. ANS:A   Obstetric and Gynecologic Surgery
45. ANS:C   Obstetric and Gynecologic Surgery
46. ANS:A   Obstetric and Gynecologic Surgery
47. ANS:C   Obstetric and Gynecologic Surgery
48. ANS:C   Obstetric and Gynecologic Surgery
49. ANS:B   Ophthalmic Surgery
50. ANS:B   Ophthalmic Surgery
51. ANS:B   Otorhinolaryngologic Surgery
52. ANS:A   Otorhinolaryngologic Surgery

53. ANS:C   Otorhinolaryngologic Surgery

54. ANS:A   Otorhinolaryngologic Surgery

55. ANS:D   Otorhinolaryngologic Surgery

56. ANS:B   Otorhinolaryngologic Surgery

57. ANS:D   Oral and Maxillofacial Surgery

58. ANS:B   Oral and Maxillofacial Surgery

59. ANS:B   Oral and Maxillofacial Surgery

60. ANS:B   Oral and Maxillofacial Surgery

61. ANS:C   Plastic and Reconstructive Surgery

62. ANS:A   Plastic and Reconstructive Surgery

63. ANS:C   Plastic and Reconstructive Surgery

64. ANS:B   Plastic and Reconstructive Surgery

65. ANS:B   Plastic and Reconstructive Surgery

66. ANS:B   Plastic and Reconstructive Surgery

67. ANS:D   Plastic and Reconstructive Surgery

68. ANS:D   Genitourinary Surgery

69. ANS:C   Genitourinary Surgery

70. ANS:A   Genitourinary Surgery

71. ANS:C		Genitourinary Surgery
72. ANS:C		Genitourinary Surgery
73. ANS:C		Orthopedic Surgery
74. ANS:D		Orthopedic Surgery
75. ANS:C		Orthopedic Surgery
76. ANS:A		Cardiothoracic Surgery
77. ANS:B		Cardiothoracic Surgery
78. ANS:C		Cardiothoracic Surgery
79. ANS:B		Cardiothoracic Surgery
80. ANS:C		Cardiothoracic Surgery
81. ANS:B		Cardiothoracic Surgery
82. ANS:C		Peripheral Vascular Surgery
83. ANS:C		Peripheral Vascular Surgery
84. ANS:B		Peripheral Vascular Surgery
85. ANS:C		Peripheral Vascular Surgery
86. ANS:B		Peripheral Vascular Surgery
87. ANS:C		Peripheral Vascular Surgery
88. ANS:B		Neurosurgery

89. ANS:D   Neurosurgery

90. ANS:B   Neurosurgery

91. ANS:D   Neurosurgery

92. ANS:A   Neurosurgery

93. ANS:C   Neurosurgery

94. ANS:C   Neurosurgery

95. ANS:A   Neurosurgery

96. ANS:C   Physical Environment and Safety Standards

97. ANS:C   Physical Environment and Safety Standards

98. ANS:B   Physical Environment and Safety Standards

99. ANS:C   Physical Environment and Safety Standards

100. ANS:C   Physical Environment and Safety Standards

101. ANS:D   Physical Environment and Safety Standards

102. ANS:D   Asepsis and Sterile Technique

103. ANS:A   Asepsis and Sterile Technique

104. ANS:B   Asepsis and Sterile Technique

105. ANS: D   Asepsis and Sterile Technique

106. ANS: D   Standards of Conduct

107. ANS:B   Standards of Conduct

108. ANS:A   Standards of Conduct

109. ANS:D   Standards of Conduct

110. ANS:D   Standards of Conduct

111. ANS:D   Standards of Conduct

112. ANS:B   Standards of Conduct

113. ANS:C   Standards of Conduct

114. ANS:C   Standards of Conduct

115.   ANS: B   Principle's of Human Anatomy

116.   ANS: D Principle's of Human Anatomy

117.   ANS: C   Principle's of Human Anatomy

118.   ANS: C   Principle's of Human Anatomy

119. ANS: D   Principle's of Human Anatomy

120.   ANS: C Principle's of Human Anatomy

121.   ANS: A Principle's of Human Anatomy

122.   ANS: C Principle's of Human Anatomy

123. ANS: E   Principle's of Human Anatomy

124. ANS: B   Principle's of Human Anatomy

125. ANS: A Principle's of Human Anatomy

126. ANS: B Principle's of Human Anatomy

127. ANS: C Principle's of Human Anatomy

128. ANS: C Principle's of Human Anatomy

129. ANS: E Principle's of Human Anatomy

130. ANS: B Principle's of Human Anatomy

131. ANS: A Principle's of Human Anatomy

132. ANS: C Principle's of Human Anatomy

133. ANS: A Principle's of Human Anatomy

134. ANS: A Principle's of Human Anatomy

135. ANS: A Principle's of Human Anatomy

136. ANS: C Principle's of Human Anatomy

137. ANS: C Principle's of Human Anatomy

138. ANS: D Principle's of Human Anatomy

139. ANS: C Principle's of Human Anatomy

140. ANS: D Principle's of Human Anatomy

141. ANS: D Principle's of Human Anatomy

142. ANS: B Principle's of Human Anatomy

143.   ANS: A Principle's of Human Anatomy

144. ANS: A   Principle's of Human Anatomy

145.   ANS:C Asepsis and Sterile Technique

146. ANS: B   Asepsis and Sterile Technique

147. ANS: C   Asepsis and Sterile Technique

148. ANS: D   Asepsis and Sterile Technique

149. ANS: B   Asepsis and Sterile Technique

150. ANS: A   Asepsis and Sterile Technique

151. ANS: B   Asepsis and Sterile Technique

152. ANS: D   Asepsis and Sterile Technique

153. ANS: A   Asepsis and Sterile Technique

154. ANS: B   Asepsis and Sterile Technique

155. ANS: C   Surgical Pharmacology and Anesthesia

156. ANS: D   Surgical Pharmacology and Anesthesia

157. ANS: A   Surgical Pharmacology and Anesthesia

158. ANS: D   Surgical Pharmacology and Anesthesia

159. ANS: B   Surgical Pharmacology and Anesthesia

160. ANS: B   Surgical Pharmacology and Anesthesia

161. ANS: B	Surgical Pharmacology and Anesthesia

162. ANS: C	Surgical Pharmacology and Anesthesia

163. ANS: B	Surgical Pharmacology and Anesthesia

164. ANS: D	Asepsis and Sterile Technique

165. ANS: A	Asepsis and Sterile Technique

166. ANS: B	Asepsis and Sterile Technique

167. ANS: A	Asepsis and Sterile Technique

168. ANS: B	Asepsis and Sterile Technique

169. ANS: A	Asepsis and Sterile Technique

170. ANS: C	Asepsis and Sterile Technique

171. ANS: A	Asepsis and Sterile Technique

172. ANS: D	Asepsis and Sterile Technique

173. ANS: B	Surgical Pharmacology and Anesthesia

174. ANS: C	Surgical Pharmacology and Anesthesia

175. ANS: A	Surgical Pharmacology and Anesthesia